"This book is a distillation of five decades of experience combining a psychological perspective with a hand-on pragmatic approach to treating drug dependence. Besides having taught at NYC Metropolitan Area colleges, hospitals and professional schools, he has a long-time NYC Metropolitan Area private practice. Overall, this book should be a valuable resource for those working in the field of substance abuse treatment and rehabilitation."

—*Anthony F. Philip, Ph.D*

"Wonderful ability to utilize psychodynamic principles in his therapeutic work with those individuals who are mired in the downward spiral of addiction."

—*Richard A. Winters, M.D., Psychiatrist*

".. a fearless therapist. Willing to take on the most difficult case and find hope..."

—*Daniel Mierlak, M.D., Ph.D.*

"Al Borrelli has been a fine mentor and colleague of mine for the past several years. He is a true scholar in the field, with an unsurpassed wealth of knowledge in his areas of expertise. From his extensive training in psychoanalytic theory, substance abuse treatment, and EMDR, he has developed a most comprehensive approach to treatment reflective of his deep understanding of human suffering and how best to alleviate it. His passion for his work, compassion, and scientific zeal are inspirational."

—*Dan Edelman, Psy.D.*

"I met Al Borrelli in 1994 and he quickly earned my confidence as a gifted diagnostician and therapist. Over the next twenty years I worked closely with Al, collaborating with him in the treatment of individuals with both Mental Health and co-occurring Substance Abuse Use Disorders. He has proven to be the key to successful treatment for some of my most challenging patients. His therapeutic skills are well honed and founded on evidence-based models of treatment. However, the most valuable skill he brings to his practice is the ability to use a wide array of psychological tests to establish accurate diagnoses. Before beginning treatment with therapy or medication, I've come to rely on his expertise as a master diagnostician."

—*Jeffrey A. Berman, M.D., FASAM*
Diplomate, American Board of Psychiatry and
Neurology (ABPN)

THE MATCH

THE MATCH

ACADEMIC/APPLIED PSYCHOLOGY AND
THE CHEMICAL DEPENDENCE FIELD:
A PARALLEL HISTORY OF THEORY,
ASSESSMENT, AND TREATMENT

ALFRED A. BORRELLI

FCP

Full Court Press
Englewood Cliffs, New Jersey

Published in the United States of America
by Full Court Press, 601 Palisade Avenue,
Englewood Cliffs, NJ 07632
fullcourtpressnj.com

ISBN 978-1-938812-95-8
Library of Congress Catalog No. 2017947603

*Editing and book design by Barry Sheinkopf for Bookshapers
(bookshapers.com)*

Cover art by Ismael Perez

ACKNOWLEDGMENTS

I have written this work in part to honor my forebears—my paternal grandparents, Elias and Ermelinda, and maternal grandparents, Vincent and Margaret, all of whom had great respect for education.

My parents, Al and Ann, were highly supportive; my mother for anything I wished to do, and my father who surrendered his desire to become a physician to support his family of origin, and in wanting me to achieve whatever I could.

My wife Carmela's support included an unqualified love for me, without which I would have lived a very different life.

Lastly, Anthony F. Philip, Ph.D., Diplomate, A.B.P.P., was my professor in graduate school and has been my psychoanalyst and mentor all of my life. I owe him the debt of providing the model of a clinical psychologist for me to emulate.

TABLE OF CONTENTS

FOREWORD

ALTHOUGH THE PURPOSE OF THIS BOOK is to inform, it has never been to applaud myself. Those who know me know I do not have pride in myself; I am merely satisfied that I attempt to complete what I set out to do, the same goal I have for my children.

My mission has been to honor my wife Carmela and those before me—my parents and grandparents on the one hand, and colleagues, my students, practitioners, and academicians on the other.

Prominent among these is Anthony F. Philip, Ph.D. I met him in graduate school, subsequent to his post-graduate training in psychoanalysis at Austin Riggs Institute in Stockbridge, Massachusetts.

He stood out from other professors in his appearance and style but mostly, and more importantly, in his being—his presence. I found his calm and *center* admirable and worthy of developing in myself, if I did not already possess it.

I was on the teaching faculty at New York Medical College, CCNY (City College of New York), and UMDNJ (University of Medicine and Dentistry of New Jersey), as well as other medical and psychological faculties, while working toward my doctorate in psychology at the Graduate Faculty of The New School For Social Research in New York City, when I decided to enter psychoanalysis with him.

Thus began a six-and-a half-year process of three times per week on a couch at Columbia that provided me with greater stability, insight, and empathy than I had. This experience, as well as Tavistock weekends recommended by him, had the greatest impact on my career. It changed who I was and how I viewed my life in ways not possible without it. I am hopeful I have served his tutelage well.

I have envisioned this book for decades, holding virtually all its information in my head. After fifty years of work in the field of psychology, and slightly less in addiction, it was time to think and write, to compose a framework for the development of ideas in both fields to pass on to others.

This book is designed primarily for professionals in mental health and addictions, and only secondarily for those outside this field such as recovering personnel in treatment settings.

Since my training is mostly within psychology, specifically clinical and some experimental, as well as biology, I have a tendency to view issues from these vantage points. It would be easy for others to claim this is a bias, but I would exercise caution, since well-reasoned arguments with evidence stand on their own.

There is a penchant in psychologically oriented fields to attribute everything to "mental forces" somehow separated from biological roots. Freud was the father of psychoanalysis and, perhaps indirectly, clinical psychology as well. As a neurologist, from the beginning he believed biology ruled the roost. My view is even more strident; without the brain, nothing happens and therefore nothing exists.

Simply put, "ontogeny recapitulates phylogeny"; we are whom we come from. More precisely, we are a product of the familial interaction of nature and nurture; however, it seems over time that the balance of influence has moved in favor of biology and nature.

In spite of often wide individual differences, we are all more alike than otherwise. All of us are mortal, and all are able to see, hear, and sense only part of the spectrum of colors and objects, for example.

As an example, it seems counterintuitive to us to accept the truth that microscopic neutrons can pass through our bodies without us knowing, feeling, or seeing them, but it is so. Some things are too small for us to perceive and remain high mysteries for the average observer.

Applying postulates from clinical psychology to the early addiction field was natural for me, so this treatise reflects that. The field of addiction, when I entered it, was an amalgam of seat–of–the-pants principles derived by recovering people designed to change an addict's behavior. To the extent this was an honest enterprise, it was practical but psychologically naive and professionally uninformed, by definition.

Its shortcomings as a set of principles are not to be derided, because they helped, and continue to help, many people who had little or no success with other approaches from professionals who at that time knew little about addiction, and essentially forced it to fit their conceptions of human behavior and mental health.

Mental health professionals' naiveté was present here as well in their expectation that the addict would be as honest in wanting help from psychological and psychiatric professionals as were their neurotic patients.

There was therefore a need for mental health professionals to apply their principles to addiction tempered by the recovering addict's practical knowledge. This was easier in theory than reality. The degree of suspicion on both groups' parts was intractable at times.

From the beginning it seemed improvements could be made, but only after rapport and trust were established.

My observations led to viewing the analytic, cognitive, and behavioral concepts as fitting many areas of addiction treatment. I have attempted to explain what I have learned and done over the past five decades.

But before delving into this project, it was necessary to present and resolve the differences in traditional psychology from its beginning to the present.

Essentially, psychological theories of human behavior all of course made different assumptions, but there were overlaps in processes or even similarities in representation with merely different names for these "differences." If they are placed side by side, a somewhat unified theory appears, and the compilation of variations at any given time in a science's history is then somewhat derivable.

Instead of applying techniques from one field, it was preferable to apply what worked best for a particular issue. While most of psychology can be learned and applied without oneself being psychoanalyzed, most practitioners entered psychoanalysis to resolve their own issues and to avoid having those issues color their interpretations of their patients' behaviors.

So we have a system of ideas that, when applied to others' problems, would be different if the practitioner were or were not an acolyte of psychoanalysis. In the early days of the government-supported addiction field—the 1960s—psychoanalysis was still in its heyday.

My approach was formed by analysis at Columbia, as well as by my understanding of what I learned and taught at places like the City College of New York (CCNY), New York Medical College, and the University of Medicine and Dentistry of New Jersey (UMDNJ). Thus, I saw human behavior and other psychological theories through the lens of psychoanalysis, as well as other systems.

My doctoral-level training at the Graduate Faculty of the New School For Social Research was overwhelmingly cognitive and, specifically, Gestalt. The term "New School" in fact represents the new cognitive psychology from Germany in the persons of Wertheimer, Kohler, Koffka, and others in the 1920s and '30s.

Once unification occurs, applying these principles and therapies to addiction is possible and provides us with more thorough, accurate, and complete treatments. The comparison again involves translation, because addiction theories, like the field itself, grew up outside the mainstream of psychological thought.

I have organized the chapters in historical sequential order, i.e., beginning with the initiation of the field of psychology with Plato's philosophy and others through the centuries, to eighteenth-century philosophy, to mental philosophy, and then to experimental psychology with Wundt. So, as has been noted, "Psychology has a long past, but a short history."

At that point there was a split between philosophy and psychology, as psychology began to develop on its own. There began a parallel course with psychology on the one hand and, about a hundred years later, the chemical dependence field on the other. In this way, one can see how the Chemical Dependence (CD) field was, and was not, affected by major changes in psychology.

We will see that the CD field held on to simpler, much less sophisticated concepts, which is only one of the problems it had and has. Resolution of the recovering addict's personal problems, which may be only somewhat related to their addiction, is another.

Becoming abstinent is easy; becoming mentally healthy is far more involved and beyond the capabilities of most recovering staff to provide, though they would likely reject this notion. This is also true of other non-mental health professional people.

Definition Of Terms

Average Expectable

When scientific discussions bear upon predictability, non-scientific and sometimes scientific individuals will employ concepts alien to the precision of the science at hand.

For example, if science uncovers a concept such as birth order— the correlation of certain behaviors correlative to one's order of birth in a family—the common conception is that it holds in all cases, i.e., the correlation is +1.00. Additionally, if the eldest is regarded as usually more intelligent, then *all* first-borns must be more intelligent and, if not, "The theory is wrong."

Since human sciences, such as psychology, rarely possess this level of precision in prediction, it is not possible to employ the man-on-the-street's view of science—statistics in this case. Instead, it is understood there are correlations in orders of predictability, with correlates ranging from 0 to 100, plus and minus, therefore -1.00 through 0, and then to +1.00.

In this scheme, -1.00 means the behavior discussed varies inversely with the comparison; 0 means there is no relationship between the two variables; and +1.00 means the variables have a relationship in which the presence of one always implies the presence of the other.

The absolute ends of the spectrum rarely occur in human behavior because humans are the most complex phenomenon we study in science—we are essentially studying the scientist or person who is, in turn, studying other organisms. It should also be noted that Psychology does not study just *human* behavior; the field has fifty-six divisions.

Since the environment and the organism acting within it rarely co-vary in mathematically precise ways, we need a term that accounts for this loose or "fuzzy logic" relationship. Heinz Hartmann, the famous psychoanalyst, employed the term "average expectable" to correct simplistic interpretations of complex data.

So when a concept or series of concepts is posited, there is the understanding that the organism and/or environment are within a "normal" or "average expectable" varying setting, and that the relationship is only approximated.

The next level of the non-scientific argument involves a similar issue—genetics—or "DNA *vs.* Environment." In science, there again is no postulation of "this or that." It is a loose combination of both entities interacting together in varying percentages.

For example, if a man inherits DNA, that makes it more probable he will inherit CVAs (cardiovascular accidents), but it does *not* mean he will inherit the DNA *expression*, since each of us carries all the DNA of all of our ancestors but express only a small part. If he did, it would not mean the CVA would *definitely* occur, since the environment plays a greater or lesser moderating role, including exercise, diet, and medicines in this case.

With regard to alcohol/drug DNA, the case is similar. Firstly, there is rarely a single gene responsible for a complex array of human behaviors. We may only *know* of one gene at a particular time, but this does not mean that is all there is.

Secondly, the only fairly firm interpretation to make is that the presence of familial genetic factors makes it *more likely* the disease will occur and that the disease will be *more intractable*.

Consider the Bio-Diagnostic or Parity (with medical treatment) aspects of insurance plans. If a syndrome is heritable, then treatment can employ unlimited sessions, since it is more difficult and time-consuming to treat. Thus, psychological issues are treated as physical ones; within reason, the number of sessions is not tightly controlled but evaluated from time to time for medical necessity.

Over-Determination

Again, from the field of psychoanalysis, Erik Erikson, in *Childhood and Society* (1953) postulated that all behaviors are over-determined. To avoid the overly simplified theoretical postulates that make human behavior the result of one or two factors and at the same level of efficacy, this term broadens the issue.

For example, if a large adult individual cowers in front of his parents, who are reprimanding him, we can assume his aversion is, for example, the result of moral/behavioral standards, or abuse, but we may be oversimplifying.

If, instead, we posit that his aversive behavior is the result of *many* factors, then these may include his moral standards, his fear of physical confrontations with his parents or anybody, his illusory view under the influence of chemicals, his psychotic representation of them, his fear of his own responsive anger, etc., and that whichever or all of these factors is operating, they may be at varying strength levels as well, then we are far closer to representing the complexity of human behavior *outside* the lab—a *major* difference in psychological/psychiatric theorizing.

Factor Analysis

Mathematical representations of human behavior are made in several fields of endeavor, not just psychology. The difference, however, lies in the degree of sophistication, a matter I will pursue in later chapters. The point to make here is that human behavior is not predictable as a one-to-one ratio, as noted earlier with correlation.

Additionally, factor analysis is of course far more involved and accurate than correlation, but it represents *factors* or *aspects* of behavior that contribute to larger behavior complexes. It is similar to over-determination above, but with measured precision.

A behavioral complex of love, e.g., could be composed of factors such as: affiliation .35, intimacy .45, and sexual attraction .77, not adding up to 100 because each factor is on its own 0-100 scale.

Zeitgeist

The German word for "spirit" is used in science to represent the occasional situation in which two or more investigators reach the same or essentially the same conclusions/insights without knowing of each other's work. The assumption is, the ideas are "in the air" and anyone could pick them up.

There are many such coincidences, and Thomas S. Kuhn's *The Structure of Scientific Revolutions* (1962) makes many of them clear. We will discuss this very issue, as well as the book, later.

Goal of Attempted Resolution

I hope this introduction elucidates the main ideas to be discussed. In short, my goal is to provide extensive information about psychology, biology, addiction, and medicines.

The secondary goal is to blend apparently disparate theories and issues to provide a more effective manner of viewing life in general, and improving the lives of chemically dependent people.

Chapter One

"PSYCHOLOGY HAS A LONG PAST
BUT A SHORT HISTORY"

T HE BABYLONIANS, THROUGH PHILOSOPHY, were the first to localize specific sensory and motor functions. Later, the Egyptians performed brain surgery to change behavior, making clear their assumption that the brain was the seat of the mind" (Klein, 1970, p. 3).

Psychology as a formal field did not exist prior to the mid-1800s and began only as an experimental, not clinical, approach with Wilhelm Wundt's laboratory in 1851.

"The first writings containing inquiries of a 'psychological' type occur in Aristotle, but primarily in Plato, who seems to have pre-empted Freud with some ideas" (pp. 291-303). Also, "The word 'psychology' did not appear in the title of a book until the 16th century" (p. 55).

Klein states, "What Plato described in terms of an irrational soul, Freud described in terms of the unconscious, the amoral id or the dynamism of repression" (p. 55).

As Klein notes, there are many other parallels between the two great thinkers, and it appears that Brentano's years of medical school lectures to Freud also included references to philosophy and Plato.

Leibnitz, Locke, and Schopenhauer anticipated some of Freud's notions in the 1900s. In fact, Klein noted that Spinoza stated "men's desires and unconscious motivation" a hundred years before Freud (1970, p. 408). The concept of the Zeitgeist, that certain ideas are "in the air," does not apply here, however, because these aspects are *not contemporaneous.*

Atomistic Analysis vs. Holism

Democritus lived in the time of Plato and began the historical discussion of Atomism (Klein, 1970, p. 64). Much later, in the eighteenth century, John Locke held the view that experience is made of elements of sensation that could combine over time to become organized patterns and perceptions. This idea has continued over time to provide behaviorists with "elements" of their formulae.

Locke, and those who followed him, faced the same dilemma: "It finds in sensation the last product of analysis and then makes it the first element of construction" (Brett, 1912, p. 150).

Plato held that experience is holistic and, in his opinion, probably inborn. In the twentieth century, the Gestaltists maintained that experience is not composed of elements, but the organism views it as a whole—from the beginning of the percept.

One can view this duality from two thousand years ago as a continuing struggle for the truth, of course. I think the holistic view is closer to reality, but investigators were then looking at different aspects of a percept. As always, these theories are not mutually exclusive.

You can see elements, if you wish to see only "building blocks," as (JNDs) Just Noticeable Differences, derived from Ernst Weber's later involvement in experimental psychology (Fancher & Rutherford, 2012, pp. 167-171).

Weber's Law involves a person, e.g., adjusting a sound or light next to a constant sound or light and telling the experimenter when the adjusted light or sound is *just noticeably different from the first.* This difference, expressed as a percentage or decimal, is a constant for Weber.

It is also possible to see the wholes as pictures of the full experience. The key question is not whether one or the other dominates—they probably both do at different times, and in different situations, depending upon how the particular person *perceives* the total of their reality. It is the type of brain that matters initially and consistently and that accounts for most of the variance, in my opinion.

In my view, this involves more than the duality of percepts in lab work but also includes the genetic differences among individuals that control their perceptions about everything—more about this later.

"[Freud's] predecessors from Plato to Hegel may have anticipated some of his insights, but neither they nor their followers grasped the implications sufficiently to work them out as Freud did" (Klein, 1970, p. 67).

Philosophy To Scientific Philosophy
To Academic Psychology

Philosophy at the time of Locke, Spinoza, Leibnitz, and others continued the tradition of Plato in examining the human mind and theorizing about elements and wholes. At some point in the eighteenth century, psychology, in its embryonic state, began the scientific tradition with Just Noticeable Difference (JND), an elemental, atomistic notion.

Wilhelm Wundt was the architect of the new enterprise of Experimental Psychology. *Clinical* psychology was about a hundred years away from its beginning, and Freud was, indirectly, to be its father. The process of measuring human behavior in this more precise experimental way with smaller segments of behavior continued the elemental atomistic tradition of some philosophers. It also set the stage for behavioristic psychology and today's "evidence-based" theorizing with cognitive behavioral psychology.

In the late 1800s, parallel to Wundt's experimentation, Freud had a mentor in psychiatry, Jean Martin Charcot, who specialized in hypnosis as a means of treating hysteria.

The approach intrigued Freud, because it represented an entry into the mind other than by the conscious route. Later, he noted hypnosis blocked the mind and pushed psychic material further away—an idea not fully embraced to this day.

Experimental Psychology–Wilhelm Wundt

Wundt established the first *experimental* lab and thereby set off the new psychology from philosophy proper, even though some philosophers, since Plato at least, had entertained mental notions similar to psychology as later practiced.

It is interesting that philosophy did not *end* abruptly, and that psychology did not *begin* abruptly. The parallel course between the two fields continued for over two thousand years, so far.

It is the laboratory setting that made psychology a measurable, quantifiable field of study that split it off from the more subjective theorizing of philosophy. This is Wundt's major gift to the field of psychology and the history of ideas.

Gustav Fechner's Just Noticeable Difference (JND) notion of studying perception and registering the fractionations of the conscious experience of subjects was the beginning of experimentation for Wundt.

Wundt's goal was to study the elements of percepts, and he attempted to define the structure of atomism, which we have seen before in philosophy, and this continued the path of study toward behaviorism, which blossomed in the twentieth century.

Curiously, Wundt was not a total adherent of Atomism; even though he searched for elements, he had a more holistic approach—one closer to Plato and Freud. Wundt's theory of the mind was known as "Structuralism," and he trained people to introspect. Over time it became clear there was not enough internal agreement among "introspectors," so subjectivity became a problem.

Classical Psychoanalysis-Freud

Freud experienced his theoretical assumptions via his own dreams, which led him to classical psychoanalysis. The first issue involves correcting this notion, still held by many lay people and professionals, even in psychology and psychiatry. Most students and professionals assume there are only two versions of classical psychoanalysis, and that both are only clinical.

However, there are four versions, and two types-clinical and academic (Rappaport, 1960). This notion makes discussions about

The Field much more complex. If we are in search of the truth, completeness counts.

For some time we have also dealt with psychoanalysis as a wave of the past, which it is, but also as a one-line footnote, which it is not. This is our second issue.

In brief, the first of the four versions involved the conscious–unconscious split, explaining how ideas and motives we experience have two levels, with one very much outside our purview yet influencing our conscious mind. Dreams, as Freud later stated in *Interpretation of Dreams* (1913, p. 55), were "The royal road to the unconscious."

Freud experienced and theorized the unconscious as a vast area of our life–much more so than others before him who also knew of the unconscious and its effects. In the process, he noted the unconscious "spoke" in symbols, its own language, that required *interpretation*-and this is the second version.

The third version of psychoanalysis involved the concepts of id, ego, and superego. The id was the repository of native, hidden, drive states (e.g., love–hate); the ego was, initially, roughly parallel to the conscious self; and the superego was the moral arbiter of the mind, at least in its earliest expression. In a later version, the ego had unconscious aspects.

This version also included ego-enhancing events and the constitutional (genetic and "genetic") aspects of the undifferentiated ego. This set of ideas was developed further by Heinz Hartmann, who theorized in the 1900s, and developed the term "average expectable."

The fourth version was found in Freud's posthumous writings— the pre-undifferentiated ego and cultural influences in which the ego had two aspects—the genetic and the experienced. The person then had inherited elements as well as those influenced by their environment.

Margaret Mead

Freud's view here paralleled the new "ego-psychoanalytic" theory espoused by Erik Erikson (1953) and others, and addressed Margaret Mead's anthropological view that the sexually repressed culture was not universal, and that Freud's conception of the individual's intrapsychic functioning was not the whole story.

As an aside, while true, Mead's finding of a few primitive cultures that did not support Freud's universal assumption of repression and other psychic forces never seemed terribly germane to the entire psychoanalytic enterprise, since even she would have agreed that his theories covered all else. Other psychoanalysts who suggested alternate nurturing contexts were Jung, Adler, Horney, and Rank.

Erik Erikson

Erik Erikson, in *Childhood and Society* (1953), spoke of "triple bookkeeping"—somatic factors, social context, and ego development. In this way, all behaviors had dimensions to them at all times. This was "over-determination," multiple factors at multiple levels of influence. It is clear this type of theorizing differs greatly from philosophically based and early experimental lab based theories, a point we will see continuing into the future.

The general trend in psychoanalysis—by Erikson's time, the 1950s—changed in another way: *He was theorizing development beyond adolescence and adding stages into old age, as well as adding a social aspect to Freud's stages of the individual's development.*

Beyond these theoretical issues, there was the point made by David Rapaport in his monograph *The Structure of Psychoanalytic Theory* (1960), that the academic aspect of psychoanalytic theory was only half of it—the clinical portion was separate, and the validity of one did not affect the validity of the other.

Assuming dreams were the access to our unconscious was only the first step in analyzing our drives and motivations; they had to be interpreted. Then, as now, there are those who believed differently from Freud.

Carl Jung was Freud's peer in psychoanalysis and theorized about universal "archetypes," which were pictures carried in our genes. Physiological genes were of course unknown at the time, and the term was merely a heuristic device that represented our conscious and unconscious lives. Archetypes were one of the concepts that led to a split between him and Freud.

Jung began the field of "analytical psychology" and believed spirituality was an integral part of our lives and personality. Serendipitously, this led to his interest in Alcoholics Anonymous, which he helped to establish. This connection is probably the first juncture between the broader field of psychology and the field of addiction.

Personality Theories

I have chosen a small sample from the legion of personality theories available to provide evidence of the sophistication, even genius, of those professionals who were and are mostly psychologists.

I also want to make clear that those outside the mental health field are employing naive and ineffective treatment techniques with no scientific evidence for patient improvement.

Philosophic assumptions involved Freedom versus Determinism, Heredity versus Environment, Uniqueness versus Universality, Active versus Reactive, and Optimistic versus Pessimistic.

What is personality? Is there such a concept as personality style that was dominant in 1950s–1970s?

In 1937, Gordon Allport described two ways to study personality:

Nomothetic "seeks general laws applied to many different people, such as self-actualization or extraversion.

Idiographic "attempts to understand the unique aspects of a particular individual."

"The major theories include: trait perspective, type, psychodynamic, humanistic, biological, behaviorist, and social learning perspective" (Allport, 1937, p. 211).

Chapter Two

GLOBAL VERSUS SPECIFIC THEORIES

I N THE EARLY DAYS OF THE PSYCHOLOGY FIELD—the late 1800s— the bifurcation of the field began to occur, beginning with academic psychology, derived from the field of mathematics and later statistics, with Helmholtz and Thorndike, and concepts as Just Noticeable Difference. These were focusing on small behaviors, because they were more easily measurable in laboratories.

Control/measurement was deemed more valuable than broader concepts that were closer to everyday life but were less measurable. The goal was to build a personality theory from smaller, more exact elements.

The global approach of grand theories represented by Freud and others, by contrast, grew out of the philosophy field in part. So their concepts began, not in laboratories, but in real life, including those of Freud's patients, who were neurotic and required working backwards from their illness to its etiology. One can easily see that these two divergent approaches could lead to divergent ends that never met.

There is a parallel in many other fields—physics with planet movements, the Big Bang vs. waves and particles, and, in medicine, with "humors" vs. microbes.

The parallel view in psychology and other behavioral health fields is different from physics and medicine in that they started with large concepts, specifically from philosophy, and worked downward to smaller ones.

The larger *and* smaller aspects of physical bodies became part of a whole, and these parts met. In psychology, they did not, because the elements did not possess characteristics of physical, more easily measurable elements as they did in physics.

We still don't know if psychology and other behavioral sciences do, or can, possess building blocks that are quantifiable elements and wholes, as physics does. An even more significant issue is unique to psychology and behavioral sciences—the observer is evaluating complex humans in the only way possible, *through himself*.

In quantum physics, there is Heisenberg's Uncertainty Principle . It postulates, "There are no states that describe a particle with a definite position and a definite momentum." His dictum was, "The more precise the position, the less precise the momentum" (Jha, 2013, p. 1). For psychological interventions and measurements, the person measuring inexorably becomes a part of the equation, *and perhaps a hindrance to its solution.*

There are not only issues with observer–subject problems like those noted above; there are also pre-programmed genetic predilections that control direction.

Since Skinner, theories of human behavior have become smaller and more accurate but not more useful for explaining larger behavioral systems like language, though that was the hope and the promise. Though Skinner's system of operant conditioning could develop into a more valuable heuristic, it may never have, and then it ended its influence.

Those researchers who disagreed about its positive influence included Terwilliger (1968) and Chomsky (1968).

A different version of psychological theory—cognitive theory—-also took its place in the pantheon of psychological explanatory devices, unfortunately and mostly at the expense of discarding the unconscious–the repository of every human experience. Every theory pays a price for such drastic alterations presented as "better."

Specific Personality Theories: Trait and Type Theories

Prior to reading the following information, there is another source to consider which is very readable and explains theories within the context of personality and its situations (Ewen, 2010).

A *TRAIT* is a characteristic pattern of behavior or conscious motive that can be self-assessed or assessed by peers.

The term *TYPE* is used to identify a certain collection of traits that make up a broad general personality classification.

Trait theorists include Gordon Allport, Raymond Cattell-Hans Eysenck (Factor Analysis), Lewis Goldberg (Big Five), and John Holland (RIASEC).

Gordon Allport

Gordon Allport's trait theory "proposed that an individual's conscious motives and traits better describe personality than does that person's unconscious motivation" (Winters, 2013, pp. 276-283). He identified three types of traits:

Cardinal Traits, such as a tendency to seek out the truth (and) govern the direction of one's life.

Central Traits, which operate in daily interactions, as illustrated by a tendency to always try to control a situation.

Secondary Traits, such as a tendency to discriminate against older people, involve response to a specific situation.

The following trait theories were preceded by Sir Francis Galton's work in 1884, when he composed a list of thousands of words describing behavior.

Raymond Cattell

According to Cattell, there is a continuum of personality traits. In other words, each person contains all of these sixteen traits to a certain degree, but they might be high in some traits and low in others. The following personality trait list describes some of the descriptive terms used for each of the sixteen personality dimensions described by Cattell.

Abstractedness: Imaginative versus practical

Apprehension: Worried versus confident

Dominance: Forceful versus submissive

Emotional Stability: Calm versus high strung

Liveliness: Spontaneous versus restrained

Openness to Change: Flexible versus attached to the familiar

Perfectionism: Controlled versus undisciplined

Privateness: Discreet versus open

Reasoning: Abstract versus concrete

Rule Consciousness: Conforming versus non-conforming

Self-Reliance: Self-sufficient versus dependent

Sensitivity: Tender-hearted versus tough-minded.

Social Boldness: Uninhibited versus shy

Tension: Impatient versus relaxed

Vigilance: Suspicious versus trusting

Warmth: Outgoing versus reserved

Hans Eysenck

German-born Eysenck initially believed racial differences in intelligence could be partially explained by genetic factors, which was very controversial. Later in life he switched to a view favoring greater environmental influence.

He proposed a higher organization of personality traits into three basic groups (traits plus their opposites), which he suggested constituted types:

extraversion (as opposed to introversion)

neuroticism (as opposed to emotional stability)

psychoticism (as opposed to impulse control).

Though Eysenck may have been over-emphasizing genetics, he opened the door to genetics at a time earlier than the rest of the field, except for Jung. In my view, this was more important than his accuracy in the previous argument.

Lewis Goldberg

The Big Five categories or traits of personality, also known as the Five Factor Model (FFM; see Goldberg, 1993) are:

Extraversion: This trait includes characteristics such as excitability, sociability, talkativeness, assertiveness, and high amounts of emotional expressiveness.

Agreeableness: This personality dimension includes attributes such as trust, altruism, kindness, affection, and other prosocial behaviors.

Conscientiousness: Common features of this dimension include high levels of thoughtfulness, with good impulse control and goal-directed behaviors. Those high in conscientiousness tend to be organized and mindful of details.

Neuroticism: Individuals high in this trait tend to experience emotional instability, anxiety, moodiness, irritability, and sadness.

Openness: This trait features characteristics such as imagination and insight, and those high in this trait also tend to have a broad range of interests.

It was also assumed, because these traits occur in many cultures, that they might be biologically based (Buss, 1995). Note this theory assumes its aspects are inherited, as Jung's Type theory did.

The five traits are not as predictive as the smaller ones within each category, because they are too broad. In this way we see the smaller elements of a theory are more amenable and therefore more easily measured and studied. The atomistic theory of elements, and the holistic theories of ancient times, are still represented.

Some research has been done to look into the structures of the brain and their connections to personality traits of the F.F.M. A main study was carried out by DeYoung et al. (2009). Results are as follows:

Neuroticism: negatively correlated with ratio of brain volume to remainder of intracranial volume; reduced volume in dorsomedial PFC; and a segment of left medial temporal lobe, including posterior hippocampus, increased volume in the mid-cingulate gyrus.

Extraversion: positively correlated with orbitofrontal cortex metabolism, increased cerebral volume of medial orbitofrontal cortex.

Agreeableness: negatively correlated with left orbitofrontal lobe volume in frontotemporal dementia patients, reduced volume in posterior left superior temporal sulcus, and increased volume in posterior cingulate cortex.

Conscientiousness: volume of middle frontal gyrus in left lateral PFC.

Openness to experience: No regions large enough to be significant, although the parietal cortex may be involved.

John Holland

The S.D.S. is a direct product of a theory of personality types and environmental models developed by John Holland.

The theory posits that all people can be categorized into six personality types:

- *Realistic* (R)
- *Investigative* (I)
- *Artistic* (A)
- *Social* (S)
- *Enterprising* (E)
- *Conventional* (C)

The SDS (Self-Directed Search) measures the degree to which

one resembles each of the personality types, producing a three-letter
Summary Code that expresses the complexity of a personality.

Holland's RIASEC Model

ARTISTIC

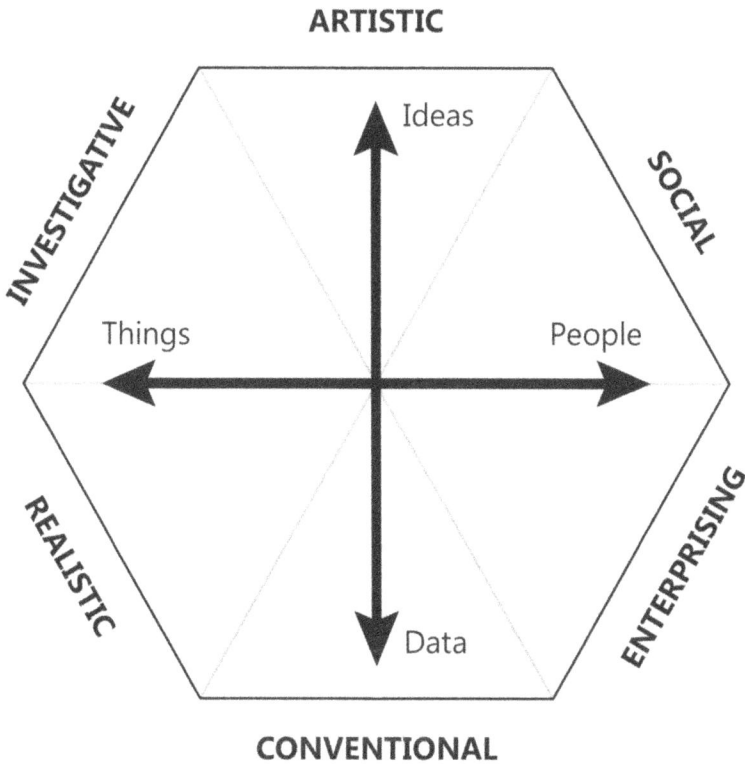

CONVENTIONAL

According to Holland's theory, the same personality types—Realistic, Investigative, Artistic, Social, Enterprising, and Conventional—also apply to work environments, and each environment
presents its own specific qualities and challenges.

Because both personalities and occupations can be classified
using the same system, you can use your three-letter Summary Code

to locate occupations (or fields of study, or leisure activities) that correspond best with your personality and thus are most likely to satisfy you.

Type Theories

Carl Jung

As noted earlier, Jung differed from Freud. The major difference is the inborn archetypes—icons that represented mankind's experiences from eons past. A twentieth-century development in test form was the Myers-Briggs Personality Test.

The MBTI (Myers-Briggs Type Indicator) was developed by those two authors and published in 1962. This test is based upon Carl Jung's typology theory (Jung, 1923).

Meyer Friedman and Ray H. Rosenman

Another twentieth-century *type* theory was developed by a cardiologist named Meyer Friedman; he and his co-theorist, Ray H. Rosenman, coined the names of personality types of those who were more prone to cardiac issues and those who were less so. The first group was Type A, and the latter, Type B.

Although both physicians knew well the physiological aspects of cardiac issues, there was doubt about the role of non-physiological factors like stress and personality.

One of the striking observations was the manner in which their waiting room chairs had worn seats, fronts, and armrests. They deduced the Type As had occupied those chairs and caused the wear by pulling themselves forward to leave the chairs and ask how much longer it would be for their appointment (McLeod, 2008, p.

1), This, however, was not the major contribution they made to the cardiology field; Type A and Type B were.

Psychoanalytic Theories

Classical psychoanalytic theory, as explained earlier, began the holistic approach in psychology, actually psychiatry, or even more accurately, neurology. Carl Jung took psychoanalytic theory in a somewhat different direction with archetypes, and assigned a greater role for inborn behaviors, in opposition to interactive inborn–environmental behaviors, as with Freud.

Classical Psychoanalysis

Psychoanalysis was the first formal psychotherapy in the world. It is possible to view those relationships, personal and professional that employ rapport and transference that led to comfort and change as therapy. However, these do not qualify as formal psychotherapy. Further, those therapies do not intend to incorporate these features, yet are under their influence.

Psychoanalysis, developed and employed by Freud, set the structure for other psychoanalysts. This approach, like the psychoanalytic theories of others, led to competition. Freud jealously guarded his ideas from change by others, most notably Jung.

It should be noted, "Freud valued psychoanalysis more as a general theory of civilization than as an individual treatment" (Jacoby, 1983, p. xi).

As the first psychoanalyst, Freud had no one to analyze him. His analysis required him to examine the conscious and unconscious aspects of his life, often prompted by the thoughts and feelings of his, mostly female, patients.

Freud's couch was the setting for analysis, and he sat behind his patients. Although this position would perhaps lead us to assume he did so to allow patients to free-associate without his visual interference, he stated otherwise. It was to avoid his having responses they would see.

Free association, as most people know by now, is the patient's associations as they occur without censorship of content. By doing so, patients began to experience analytic therapy, which, with dream interpretation, allows an examination of the conscious, pre-conscious, and unconscious areas.

The overall goal of this therapy is to uncover emotional connections among past associations and allow emotional, not intellectual, insight to occur. Intellectual insight is relatively useless because it is shallow and does not involve change. It is what too many therapists do when they see an opportunity to make a point that is not timed well enough to allow a connection associated with the opportunity for emotional change.

Additionally, it reinforces obsessive and conscious control over one's life, thereby reducing the actual goal of achieving emotional responses that lead to change.

This emphasis on emotion presaged the present day E.M.D.R. (Shapiro, 1995) which focuses on a "target" and an emotion that parallels it. Other cognitive therapies typically do not focus on emotion, but cognition.

Emotional change, on the other hand, is charged with feeling *of the type that connects with the issue at hand and permits resolution of that particular issue at that time.*

In my view, there is another aspect of this process that distinguishes most therapies from spontaneous human relationships involving rapport and empathy. It is the manner in which a therapist can share a patient's neurotic experiences, via the following metaphor.

In many therapies, the therapist observes what is happening from a distance. In my example the patient is on a roller coaster and the therapist on the ground. This degree of physical and emotional distance is not as effective an approach as being *in* the roller coaster car with the patient. It is much more real and intense for patient and therapist, as well as more effective.

The initiation of analysis engages the neurosis of the patient with the "transference" process whereby the patient transfers their neurotic aspects to the analyst. "Counter transference" occurs when the analyst transfers his issues to the patient and these must be evaluated by the analyst, because they interfere with treatment. The primary goal is resolution of the "transference neurosis"—announcing the beginning of the end of treatment.

These processes occur in virtually all known therapies, whether they are the goal of the therapist or not—and in most other systems they are not. The major problem for non-psychoanalytic therapists is the lack of resolution of these issues (analyzing the transference neurosis as the ending of therapy), because their presence is unknown or unimportant. When markers are set for change in therapy, they are different in nature from psychoanalysis, and more superficial. This difference leads to a different end result.

I was psychoanalyzed at Columbia in the 1960s and became much more aware of my issues. Once one experiences this, it is not possible to express glib phrases of assuredness about knowing what you know—a situation quite common in therapists from other systems. It is in this regard that Freud stated it is not possible for someone to investigate psychoanalysis without being psychoanalyzed.

With this beginning, he listened very carefully and allowed himself to follow feelings and thoughts with what analyst Theodor Reik (1983) said was "the third ear." To continue with Reik's interpretation of a pregnant patient's dream, in which she was in a dentist's chair and had a tooth removed, his next statement was, "Why did you not tell me that you had an abortion?"

The exact statement is in the book cited, but it is not as important as Reik's explanation of how to interpret patient communications. Reik's exchange is typical of an analyst's listening and interpreting, which require knowledge of the treatment approach and one's own psychoanalysis, as well as one's "observing ego." This is that part of our ego, or self if you will, that allows us to participate and even answer a patient while observing ourselves doing so at the same time.

This brief introduction to psychoanalysis provides a few techniques that are not present in other treatment approaches. Others to be illustrated later require a face-to-face approach with straightforward conversation and, of course, awareness of interpretation of thoughts and feelings.

The difference is the depth of interpretation moderated by the therapist's awareness of their own potentially intrusive issues, particularly previously unconscious ones, and the interference of face-to-face positioning.

Some famous analysts, e.g., Robert Langs (2004), use a face-to-face approach. In my opinion, this has the limitation of interfering with associations. Allowing the patient to be "on their own" is always a plus, since it rules out other influences and encourages independence in other areas of their lives at the same time.

Looking at a patient's face promotes their looking at the therapist's face and trying to divine what the latter thinks; sitting behind them prevents this. I think it's valuable that it can be applied to any cognitive-behavioral system as well, unless a specific technique militates against it.

I would like to address the issue of "defensiveness" or the colloquial "You're being defensive" to mean "You are purposely doing this." Analysts do not use these words as lay people or other systems therapists often do. For analysts, it is not possible for one to consciously employ this, because *all defenses are unconscious.* It is the case that a therapist who analyzes can interpret a patient's defenses and point them out, however.

Revised Psychoanalytic Theory

The course of psychoanalysis splits at this point into classical and "social" psychoanalysis. The classical portion focused on the individual, since Freud mainly had neurotic Victorian women as patients. He also kept a very tight rein on other theorists to maintain his theory's purity.

By the early twentieth century, other analysts modified Freud's theory by adding a much-needed "social" dimension.

Prominent among these were Karen Horney, Harry Stack Sullivan, and Erich Fromm; these psychoanalysts comprised the "Neo–Freudians."

Karen Horney

A psychiatrist, Horney, differed from Freud in many ways including his concepts of penis envy and Oedipal ideas. She was, essentially, the founder of Feminist Psychology and believed neurotic issues were not biologically based but a response to the environment, particularly in response to parents' treatment of their children.

She devised the following precepts (Horney, 1950):

Moving Toward People
1. The need for *affection and approval*; pleasing others and being liked by them.
2. The need for *a partner*, one whom they can love and who will solve all problems.

Moving Against People
3. The need for power; the ability to bend wills and achieve control over others—while most persons seek strength, the neurotic may be desperate for it.
4. The need to *exploit others;* to get the better of them. To become manipulative, fostering the belief that people are there simply to be used.
5. The need for *social recognition,* prestige and limelight.
6. The need for *personal admiration*—for both inner and outer qualities to be valued.
7. The need for *personal achievement;* though virtu-

ally all persons wish to make achievements, as with
No. 3, the neurotic may be desperate for achievement.

Moving Away from People

8. The need for *self-sufficiency* and independence; while most
   desire some autonomy, the neurotic may simply wish to discard other individuals entirely.
9. The need for *perfection;* while many are driven to perfect
   their lives in the form of well-being, the neurotic may dis-
   play a fear of being slightly flawed.
10. Lastly, the need to *restrict life practices* to within narrow
    borders, to live as inconspicuous a life as possible.

There is much to say about every theorist's ideas, but my purpose is only to offer the reader thumbnail versions of each representative theory. Horney provided an alternative view of
developing personalities, as did other Neo-Freudians. While she
notes her ideas came from her patients, they are remarkably parallel
to her own life experiences.

Her mother was strongly supportive of her goals in life, but her
father was "a cruel disciplinary figure" who favored her brother
Berndt. She believed Freud's idea of women having *penis envy* was
not biologically based, but a woman's response to men's achievements in life. She also proposed *womb envy* on the part of men.

As you can see, her emphasis is on environmental factors and,
more importantly, set the stage for psychoanalytic feminism—a
shortcoming of Freud's theory. On the other hand, in fairness,
Freud, like any theorist or thinker, could not develop an ingenious

formulation and at the same time cover every criticism that others may have.

Harry Stack Sullivan

Like Horney, Harry Stack Sullivan believed Freud was wrong about many things, especially in his ideas about biological roots. Sullivan's contribution to environmental influence was the notion that pathology arose from interpersonal interactions.

Sullivan postulated the defense of *selective inattention*, which allowed a person to avoid any threats, and this could develop into *non-participation*. Both defenses explained how one would maintain pathological behaviors. Both occurred before the defense of *psychological repression*.

He suggested that analysts should focus on internalized representations of one's self and what others called *schemata* (a term employed by Piaget as well). He also used the term *parataxic distortion*, a process by which the patient fantasizes the person of their interest, attributing characteristics not derived from reality.

Psychiatrists and psychoanalysts have since viewed Sullivan's work as applying new names to older psychoanalytic terms. His theory is not as developed as Horney's either. Her theoretical notions of moving toward, away, and against people are more developed than any of his. She also had superior ideas compared to Alfred Adler's "Will To Power."

I believe the Neo-Freudians as a group did not have as coherent a set of theories as Freud or Jung but fulfilled their mission of providing a legitimate alternative to classical psychoanalysis. Horney began the psychoanalytic feminist movement, which had some influence on the larger feminist movement outside psychoanalysis as well.

Although the Neo-Freudians mostly had the original mission of opposing Freud's ideas and adding a social dimension to his theories, they succeeded in replacing his theory with theirs as well.

Erik Erikson

Erikson was not a Neo-Freudian but an adherent of Freud's who knew Freud as a young man and had been an artist, not a psychoanalyst, when they met. He studied psychoanalysis and extended Freud's theories, not in the way the Neo-Freudians did, but, initially, as a coherent addition within classical psychoanalysis proper.

However, his emphasis on ego functions led to a newer branch of psychoanalysis known as *psychoanalytic ego psychology*.

His addition of the social component was far more sophisticated, and it would require a great deal of space to elaborate further. However, I will present a set of tables providing precepts side by side of Freud, Erikson, and Piaget, the last a major theorist in child development whose ideas fit well with psychoanalysis as another stage theorist.

Additionally, Lawrence Kohlberg's ideas about a child's development of morality are based upon Piaget's ideas—a companion piece, if you will. I believe that side-by-side presentations are an easier way of viewing and digesting complex ideas.

My choice of theorists who are complementary to Freud is not, in my opinion, a bias on my part, but rather a more objective approach to conserve more solid ideas having greater durability and longevity.

There are always others with alternate ideas and critiques of Freud and others, but presentation of those theorists will extend our discussion even more, and this is not meant to be a compendium of psychological theories.

A very sophisticated work on personality theory and research is John W. Livesley's (2001) *Handbook of Personality Disorders.* I recommend it for advanced psychological professionals only.

You may notice the tables parallel each theory and allow comparisons at levels of development in different areas of experience: Freud's psychoanalytic stages were developed in classical terms.

Erikson's stages not only add social stages, as Neo-Freudians attempted to do, but are more sophisticated and integrated with the original theory. Erikson's stages were consistent with Freud's as well as adding a dimension of the "work" each person must complete at each stage.

Piaget was not a mental health theorist but a psychologist and education theorist whose theory explained many issues in child development. He was a stage theorist, as were the others, and the stages involved: a child's perceptual-motor stages: sensori-motor, followed by internal operations—pre-operational, operational, and formal operational.

These deal with the child seeing and then manipulating objects in his environment. Later, they could manipulate the objects in their mind without external manipulation, then performing more sophisticated operations upon their environment, and finally to the point of internalizing all of an adult's percepts.

Lawrence Kohlberg added the child's gradual internalization of *moral* precepts from simple black-and-white judgments to more so-

Comparison of Freud, Erikson, Piaget, Kohlberg Theories

Approximate Age Ranges	Freud (Psychosexual)	Erikson* (Psychosocial)	Piaget (Cognitive)	Kohlberg (Moral)
Birth to 2 years Infancy	Oral Stage The mouth, tongue, and gums are a focus of pleasurable sensations in the baby's body, and feeding is the most stimulating activity.	Trust vs. Mistrust Babies either learn to trust that others will care for their basic needs, including nourishment, warmth, cleanliness, and physical contact, or to lack confidence in the care of others.	Sensorimotor Period Most action is reflexive. Perception of events is centered on the body. Objects are extensions of self. Acknowledges the external environment.	No Moral Development
1½ to 3 Years	Anal Stage The anus is the focus of pleasurable sensations in the baby's body, and toilet training is the most important activity.	Autonomy vs. Shame and Doubt Children learn either to be self-sufficient in many activities, including toileting, feeding, walking, exploring, and talking, or they doubt their own abilities.	Preconceptual Self-centered. Asks many questions. Explores the environment. Language development rapid. Associates words with objects.	No Moral Development
3 to 6 Years Early Childhood (Preschool)	Phallic Stage The phallus, or penis, is the most important body part, and pleasure is derived from genital stimulation. Boys are proud of their penis, and girls wonder why they don't have one. (Oedipal Conflict)	Initiative vs. Guilt Children want to undertake many adult-like activities, sometimes overstepping the limits set by parents and feeling guilty.	Preoperational Egocentric thinking diminishe Includes others in environment. Enjoys repeating words, may count to 10. Words express thoughts.	Preconventional Morality is a matter of good or bad, based on a system of punishments. 1. Punishment and obedience orientation. 2. Instrumental relativist orientation.

phisticated ones. A young child's ideas about morality are rigidly held, as in "rules" of games. Over time the child understands moral

Comparison of Freud, Erikson, Piaget, Kohlberg Theories (Cont.)

Approximate Age Ranges	Freud (Psychosexual)	Erikson* (Psychosocial)	Piaget (Cognitive)	Kohlberg (Moral)
7–11 Years Middle Childhood	Latency Not a stage but an interlude, when sexual needs are quiet and children put energy into conventional activities like schoolwork and sports.	Industry vs. Inferiority Children busily learn to be competent and productive in mastering new skills, or feel inferior and unable to do anything well.	Concrete Operations Solves concrete problemss. Begins to understand relationships such as size. Understands right and left. Cognizant of viewpoints.	Conventional Level Morality seen as following the rules of society. Tries to be "good." 1."Good boy, good girl." 2. Law-and-order orientation.
12–18 Years Adolescence	**Genital Stage** The genitals are the focus of pleasurable sensations, and the young person seeks genital stimulation and sexual satisfaction in heterosexual relationships.	**Identity vs. Role Confusion** Adolescents try to figure out, "Who am I?" They establish sexual, political, and career indentities or are confused about what roles to play.	Formal Operations Uses rational thinking. Reasoning is deductive and futuristic.	**Post-conventional** Morality consists of standards beyond specific group or authority figure. 1.The social contract orientation. 2. The universal ethical principle orientation. 3. Mystical and religious reflection.
18–40 Years Adulthood	Freud believed that the genital stage lasts through adulthood. He also said that the goal of a healthy life is "to love and work well.	**Intimacy vs. Isolation** Young adults seek companionship and love with another person or become isolated from others by fearing rejection or disappointment.		

*Although Erikson describes two extreme resolutions to each crisis, he recognizes that there is a wide range of outcomes between these extremes and that most people arrive at some middle course.

Comparison of Freud, Erikson, Piaget, Kohlberg Theories (Cont.)

Approximate Age Ranges	Freud (Psychosexual)	Erikson* (Psychosocial)	Piaget (Cognitive)	Kohlberg (Moral)
40–65 Years Middle Years		Generality vs. Stagnation Middle-aged adults contribute to the next generation by performing meaningful work, creative activities, and/or raising a family, or become stagnant and inactive		
65 Years + Late Adulthood		Identity vs. Despair Older adults try to make sense out of their lives, whether seeing life as a meaningful whole or despairing at goals never reached and questions never answered.		.

questions with less rigid and confined concepts—essentially a set of rules adapting more and more to the ever-expanding experiences of life.

In all of these stage theories there are similarities over time: inborn concepts and structures activated by environmental experiences, movement from less structured to more structured stages, and parallel stages that "fit" with each other.

However, no matter how congruent they are, they are very different from other theories that also make sense; these are merely the early, sophisticated ones. The next chapter will provide theories that are quite dissonant from these.

In many respects, as the brain develops, it changes the environment and is in turn changed by the environment. From early hominids onward, this process has been the same, and biology directed this process. It is in this manner that psychology is not "mental" but "biological," in my opinion.

Behaviorist Theories

Ivan Pavlov

Pavlov's early interest lay in becoming a priest, like his father, but that interest shifted to medicine and physiology. A specific interest was temperament and the term *transitory inhibition*—the capacity for different types of people to shut down after being overwhelmed by stimuli. He believed the rate of shutdown was inherited and controlled by different types of brains.

His most famous formulation was pairing the unconditioned stimulus (UCS), which is a natural and unlearned one, with one that *is* learned. An example from his research is salivation when presented with food. Pavlov paired the UCS with the conditioned stimulus (CS)—for example, pairing the sound of a bell (CS) with the presence of food leading to salivation (UCS). The bell then elicits salivation as though it were food. This was the first attempt to anchor learning to physiology and began the behaviorist tradition.

Edward Thorndike

Thorndike was an American-born academic psychologist who worked mainly at Columbia University. His greatest interest was in learning, but more so as part of educational pursuits.

Thorndike's theory of learning posits the following:

Learning is incremental.

Learning occurs automatically.

All animals learn the same way.

Law of effect: If an association is followed by a "satisfying state of affairs," it will be strengthened, and if it is followed by an "annoying state of affairs," it will be weakened.

Thorndike's law of exercise has two parts—the law of use and the law of disuse.

Law of use: the more often an association is used, the stronger it becomes.

Law of disuse: the longer an association is unused, the weaker it becomes.

Law of recency: The most recent response is most likely to re-occur.

Multiple response: problem solving through trial and error. An animal will try multiple responses if the first response does not lead to a specific state of affairs.

Set or attitude: Animals are predisposed to act in a specific way.

Prepotency of element: A subject can filter out irrelevant aspects of a problem and focus and respond only to significant elements of a problem.

Response by analogy: Responses from a related or similar context may be used in a new context.

Identical elements theory of transfer: This theory states that the extent to which information learned in one situation will transfer to another situation is determined by the similarity between the two situations. The more similar the situations are, the greater the amount of information that will transfer. Similarly, if the situations have nothing in common, information learned in one situation will not be of any value in the other situation.

Associative shifting: It is possible to shift any response from occurring with one stimulus to occurring with another. Associative shift maintains that a response is first made to situation A, then to AB, and then finally to B, thus shifting a response from one condition to another by associating it with that condition.

Law of readiness: a quality in responses and connections that results in readiness to act. Thorndike acknowledges that responses may differ in their readiness. He claims that eating has a higher degree of readiness than vomiting, and that weariness detracts from the readiness to play and increases the readiness to sleep. Also, Thorndike argues that a low or negative status in respect to readiness is called "unreadiness." Behavior and learning are influenced by the readiness or unreadiness of responses, as well as by their strength.

Identifiability: According to Thorndike, the identification or placement of a situation is a first response of the nervous system, which can recognize it; then connections may be made to one another or to another response, and these connections depend upon the original identification. Therefore, a large amount of learning is made up of changes in the identifiability of situations. Thorndike also believed that analysis might turn situations into compounds of features, such as the number of sides on a shape, to help the mind grasp and retain the situation, and increase their identifiability.

Availability: the ease of getting a specific response. For example, it would be easier for a person to learn to touch their nose or mouth than it would be for them to draw a line five inches long with their eyes closed.

Development of the law of effect. Thorndike's research focused on instrumental learning, which means that learning is developed from the organism doing something. For example, he placed a cat inside a wooden box. The cats used various methods trying to get out; however, it does not work until it hits the lever. Afterwards, Thorndike tried placing the cat inside the wooden box again, and this time the cat is able to hit the lever quickly and succeeded to get out of the box.

At first, Thorndike emphasized the importance of dissatisfaction stemming from failure as equal to the reward of satisfaction with success, though in his experiments and trials on humans he came to conclude that reward is a much more effective motivator than punishment. He also emphasized that the satisfaction must come immediately after the success, or the lesson will not sink in.

Thorndike has a sophisticated set of ideas that clearly differed from the psychoanalysts, whose focus was the assessment and treatment of psychiatric patients. They were also, of course, not interested in non-neurotic learning. Thorndike had followed Pavlov and provided the beginning formulations of behavioristic psychologists like Skinner and Watson.

B.F. Skinner

Skinner continued the behaviorist tradition, but in ingenious fashion. Prior theories postulated a stimulus–response presentation of the UCS/CS that led to learning via physiological state reduction. This pairing was required in all cases.

Skinner's genius was in *not* positing this rigid organism–environment interaction in which the environment provided the brain, with the other half of the learned behavior leading to learning. Skinner's system was called *Operant Conditioning* because the organism "operated" on its environment until it found the correct behavior intended by the experimenter, or the connection to solve a problem.

This change made the subject a more active partner in learning and shifted thinking to a more abstract level—much like children in Piaget's system. It also changed the brain's role toward ruling the search for information in its environment, making the brain the dominant partner; this relationship will be developed further in a later chapter.

Skinner followed Thorndike in his Law of Effect but added "reinforcers." Positive reinforcers increased the likelihood of an organism repeating the desired behavior; negative reinforcers decreased that likelihood; neutral reinforcers neither increased nor decreased the likelihood.

The "token economy" represents the implementation of tokens (coins, stars, candy, toys) as reinforcers for children in school settings. You will recognize this reward system as that used by parents and teachers for many years.

The ratio of rewards led to schedules of reinforcement, and there are too many of them to repeat for our purposes save "fixed" and "variable" types. In fixed rewards one would think the more reinforcers provided, the stronger the behavior; alternatively, the less reinforcement provided, the weaker. However, the opposite is true.

So learning and therapy practitioners need to be mindful of this difference. One of the prominent aspects of Therapeutic Communities (TCs) for CD treatment is to endlessly repeat information in the mistaken belief it will lead to stronger behaviors.

In my opinion, repetitions emphasize more concrete aspects of one's brain and make learned behaviors more superficial and more likely to be forgotten, or not employed as regularly. Any reinforcement and adopting the "correct" behavior is outside normal situations, because the resident in TCs would be punished if they didn't learn—and quickly. This idea has broad implications, as we proceed, which I will later expand upon.

One more interesting aspect about conditioning behavior and genetic structures involves language learning. When Skinner published a treatise on language learning, he expanded his ideas on reinforcement as the basis. Noam Chomsky (1978), a prominent linguist, challenged his theory. The obvious challenge came from the observation that children could not learn via reinforcement alone, or even mainly. The child could not, and did not, learn this way because the number of words is acquired in a multiplicative, not additive, manner.

That is, language was not learned gradually as research revealed. By two years of age, a child, particularly a female child, can speak 200 words, by two and a half years of age 300, a process called "the naming explosion." The basis for this explosion is the brain's "generational grammar," as Chomsky indicated.

The implied basis is a structure within the brain that is inherited and allows the child to apply the rules of grammar, not those learned solely from the environment, although the *specific* rules of grammar and words *are* learned this way.

You may recall the philosophical atomist and holistic ideas. The dual traditions appear here again, as they have now continued to do for at least two thousand years.

Cognitive Theories

Albert Bandura's Views

Bandura and other cognitivists were presaged by the Gestaltists in their opposition to the simple behaviorists' views on learning; e.g., Bandura critiqued Skinner's approach about trial-and-error learning.

One of the tenets of behaviorism is the need for the subject to participate actively in the learning environment. The organism in one of Bandura's experiments was a mouse that went through a maze also, but with the exception that this mouse was pulled in a wheeled carriage by another mouse.

The expectation was that the "pulling mouse" would learn the maze by observing and physically responding to it, but not that the "pulled mouse" would also learn the same things, though it did.

This may seem too commonsensical to need experimental verification, but it was and is necessary. The issue is that learning occurs in different ways and does not follow the rules of one theory.

Reinforcement

Pavlov and Skinner concluded that reinforcement operates without our awareness. Bandura disagreed and argued that we must be aware of reinforcement in order for it to be effective. In particular, reinforcement involves a change in our conscious anticipations: We are more likely to act in ways that we *expect* to produce rewards, and/or to avoid punishment:

The notion of "response strengthening" is, at best, a metaphor. Outcomes change behavior in humans largely through the intervening influence of thought.

Self-Reinforced Behavior

According to Bandura, our behavior is also influenced by

Response Strengthening

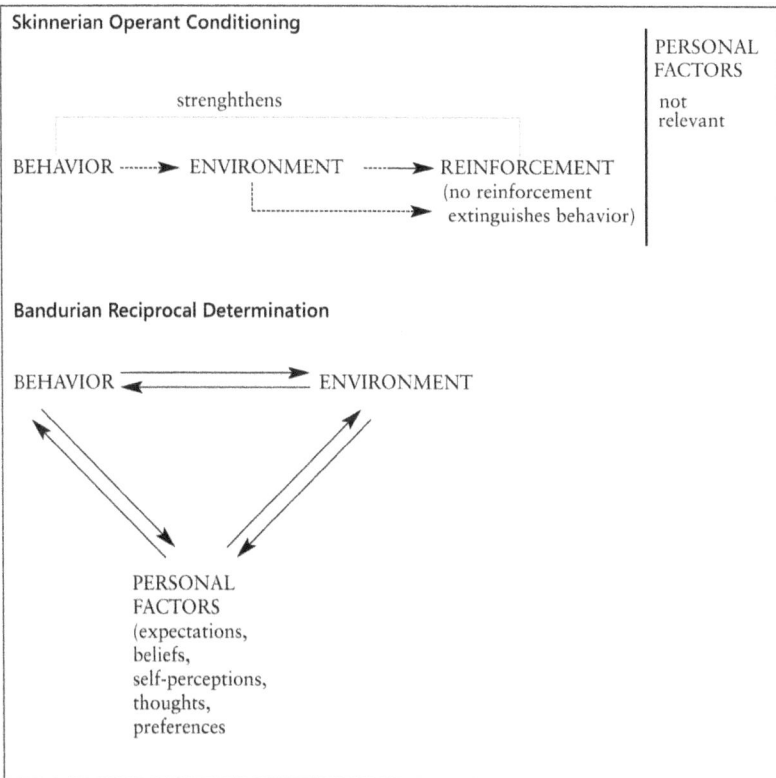

```
Skinnerian Operant Conditioning
                                                          PERSONAL
                                                          FACTORS
               strenghthens                               not
                                                          relevant
BEHAVIOR ----> ENVIRONMENT  ----> REINFORCEMENT
                                  (no reinforcement
                                   extinguishes behavior)


Bandurian Reciprocal Determination

BEHAVIOR <=======> ENVIRONMENT



         PERSONAL
         FACTORS
         (expectations,
         beliefs,
         self-perceptions,
         thoughts,
         preferences
```

Capsule Summary: Some Important Bandurian Terminology

Modeling	•A synonym for observational learning. •A form of behavior therapy wherein the client observes one or more people demonstrating desirable or effective behavior.
Observational learning (modeling, social learning)	Learning by watching other people's behavior and its consequences for them. Reinforcement is *not* necessary for observational learning to occur; but it may facilitate paying attention to the model and remembering the relevant information, or it may be essential to make the subject perform what has been learned.
Perceived self-efficacy	The extent to which a person believes that he or she can perform the behaviors required by a particular situation.
Reciprocal determinism	The continuous interrelationship of behavior, internal personal factors (e.g., thoughts, beliefs, expectations), and environmental influences, any one of which may cause any of the others.
Self-reinforcement	Establishing standards of behavior for ourselves, or prising or criticizing ourselves accordingly.
Social-cognitive theory (Social learning theory)	The name Bandura gave to his psychological theory.
Vicarious punishment	A decrease in the frequency of certain behaviors, which occurs as the result of seeing others punished or the same actions (i.e., through observational learning).
Vicarious reinforcement	An increase in the frequency of certain behaviors, which occurs as the result of seeing others rewarded for the same actions (i.e., through observational learning).

learned criteria that we establish for ourselves ("self-reinforcement"). "If actions were determined solely by external rewards and punishments, people would behave like weather vanes, constantly shifting in different directions to conform to the momentary influences impinging upon them. In actuality, people also set certain standards of behavior for themselves and respond to their own actions in self-rewarding or self-punishing ways" (Bandura, 1978, pp. 128–129, 130-158; see also Bandura, 1973, pp. 48–49; 1977, p. 67).

We then have two formulations, running parallel to each other over time, between behaviorists and cognitivists. Behaviorists believe, and have experimental evidence for, a tenet that learning occurs without a subject's awareness. Cognitivists, on the other hand, believe that learning and reinforcement can only work with awareness, and they have evidence for this position as well.

In science such apparent conundrums exist, and not because of inaccuracies in measurement or experimental design; rather, the differences are probably indicative of measuring *different processes*.

Bandura's argument also includes the notion that beliefs, attitudes, self-perceptions, etc. influence, and are influenced by, each other; Bandura called this "reciprocal determinism."

Cognitive Theorists: Perception

Herman Witkin

Witkin and others developed a theory of cognitive styles—tendencies to respond in predictable ways in various situations. The concept this group developed was Field Dependence–Field Independence.

The procedures employed to reveal one or the other, or a combination are as follows: *Rod and Frame Test; Tilting Room Test; Embedded Figures Test (EFT))* (Witkin, Karp, & Goodenough, 1962, p. 40).

Essentially, Field-Dependent subjects chose answers in these test situations by choosing information from outside their intuitive sense of vertical, and employed the givens in the environment, while the Field-Independent subjects did the reverse.

For example, In the *Rod and Frame Test,* the subject is placed in a dark room with only the visual of a lighted rod and frame, and is asked to place the rod vertically within the frame within the room; the problem is finding the true vertical to succeed.

Field Dependents are more likely to place the rod vertically within the frame without having an independent view of what is vertical within the *room.* Field Independents are more likely to operate with their own sense of the true vertical and make more correct solutions. It appears Field Independents are greater internalizers.

In the Tilting Room—Tilting Chair Test, the subject and the room can both be tilted, and this parallels the Rod and Frame Test in its orientation. The Embedded Figures Test has a series of figures within which other figures are embedded, and the subject's task is to locate them and thereby *disembed* them.

Witkin's tests were not an end in themselves but rather a means of identifying the two types of subjects and then extrapolating these styles to different life issues, like what kind of illnesses they experience (Witkin et al., 1962).

The different styles of perception are widely reflected in real world applications—e.g., my view that most CD people are Field Dependents, and chemical use/abuse make them more so. This suggests that education and therapy must consider the delivery of ideas as *dependent on the brain of the receiver.*

Walter Mischel

In 1968, Mischel published the now classic monograph *Personality and Assessment,* which created a paradigm crisis in personality psychology that changed the agenda of the field for decades. The book touched upon the problem in trait assessment that had been identified by Allport in 1937. Mischel showed that study after study failed to support the fundamental traditional assumption of personality theory that an individual's behavior with regard to a trait (e.g., conscientiousness, sociability) is highly consistent across diverse situations. Instead, Mischel's analyses revealed that the individual's behavior, when closely examined, was highly dependent upon situational cues rather than expressed consistently across diverse situations that differed in meaning. Mischel maintained that behavior is shaped largely by the exigencies of a given situation. That people act in consistent ways across different situations, reflecting an underlying consistency of personality traits, is a myth.

Situation and behavior. (See main article, Person–situation debate.) Mischel made the case that the field of personality psychology was searching for consistency in the wrong places. Instead of treating situations as the noise or "error of measurement" in personality psychology, Mischel's work proposed that, by including the situation as it is perceived by the person, and by analyzing behavior in its situational context, the consistencies that characterize the individual would be found. He argued that these individual differences would not be expressed in consistent cross-situational behavior but, instead, suggested that consistency would be found in distinctive but stable patterns of if-then, situation-behavior relations that form contextualized, psychologically meaningful "personality signatures" (e.g., "she does A when X, but B when Y").

These signatures of personality were in fact revealed in a large observational study of social behavior across multiple repeated situations over time (Mischel & Shoda, 1995). Contradicting the classic assumptions, the data showed that individuals who were similar in average levels of behavior, for example in their aggression, nevertheless differed predictably and dramatically in the types of situations in which they aggressed. As predicted by Mischel, they were characterized by highly psychologically informative if-then behavioral signatures. Collectively, this work has allowed a new way to conceptualize and assess both the stability and variability of behavior that is produced by the underlying personality system, and has opened a window into the dynamic processes within the system itself (Mischel & Ayduk, 2004, pp. 246-248).

Self-control. In a second direction beginning in the late 1960s and early 1970s, Mischel pioneered work illuminating the ability to delay gratification and to exert self-control in the face of strong situational pressures and emotionally "hot" temptations. His studies with preschoolers in the late 1960s, often referred to as "the marshmallow experiment," examined the processes and mental mechanisms that enable a young child to forgo immediate gratification and to wait instead for a larger desired but delayed reward. Continuing research with these original participants has examined how preschool delay of gratification ability links to development over the life course and may predict a variety of important outcomes (e.g., SAT scores, social and cognitive competence, educational attainment, and drug use), and can have significant protective effects against a variety of potential vulnerabilities (Mischel & Rodriguez,1989). This work also opened a route to research on temporal discounting in decision-making, and most importantly into the mental mechanisms that enable cognitive and emotional self-control, thereby helping to demystify the concept of "willpower" (Mischel & Rodriguez, 1989, pp. 933-938; Mischel & Ayduk, 2004, p. 73).

Here again, we have the opposite view of the Witkin group: inherited or given styles do not control percepts; the brain's expectations do. And yet are not the expectations partially inherited? They are, if one accepts the notion that brains have their own pre-programmed predilections; more about this in later chapters.

George Kelly

Kelly's personality theory was distinguished at the time he published the two volumes from drive theories (such as psychodynamic models) on the one hand, and behavioral theories on the other, in that people were not seen as solely motivated by instincts (such as sexual and aggressive drives) or learning history but by their need to characterize and predict events in their social world. Because the constructs people developed for construing experience have the potential to change, Kelly's theory of personality is less deterministic than drive theory or learning theory. People could conceivably change their view of the world and in so doing change the way they interacted with it, felt about it, and even others' reactions to them. For this reason, it is an existential theory, regarding humankind as having a choice to reconstrue themselves, a concept Kelly referred to as "Constructive Alternativism." Constructs provide a certain order, clarity, and prediction to a person's world. Kelly referenced many philosophers in his two volumes, but the theme of new experience being at once novel and familiar (due to the templates placed on it) is closely akin to the notion of Heraclitus: "We step and do not step in the same rivers." Experience is new but familiar to the extent that it is construed with historically derived constructs Kelly, 1955).

Constructs are bipolar categories, the way two things are alike and different from a third that people employ to understand the world. Examples of such constructs are "attractive," "intelligent," and "kind." A construct always implies contrast. So when an individual categorizes others as attractive, or intelligent, or kind, an opposite polarity is implied. This means that such a person may also evaluate the others in terms of the constructs "ugly," "stupid," or "cruel." In some cases, when a person has a disordered construct system, the opposite polarity is unexpressed or idiosyncratic. The importance of a particular construct varies among individuals. The adaptiveness of a construct system is measured by how well it applies to the situation at hand and is useful in predicting events. All constructs are not used in every situation because they have a limited range (of convenience). Adaptive people are continually revising and updating their own constructs to match new information (or data) that they encounter in their experience.

Kelly's is the only personality theory ever laid out as a testable scientific treatise with a fundamental postulate and a set of corollaries:

Fundamental postulate: "A person's processes are psychologically channelized by the ways in which he [or she] anticipates events."

· The construction corollary: "a person anticipates events by construing their replications." This means that individuals anticipate events in their social world by perceiving a similarity with a past event (construing a replication).

- The experience corollary: "a person's construction system varies as he [or she] successively construes the replication of events."
- The dichotomy corollary: "a person's construction system is composed of a finite number of dichotomous constructs."
- The organization corollary: "each person characteristically evolves, for his [or her] convenience in anticipating events, a construction system embracing ordinal relationships between constructs."
- The range corollary: "a construct is convenient for the anticipation of a finite range of events only."
- The modulation corollary: "the variation in a person's construction system is limited by the permeability of the constructs within whose range of convenience the variants lie."
- The choice corollary: "a person chooses for himself [or herself] that alternative in a dichotomized construct through which he [or she] anticipates the greater possibility for extension and definition of his system."
- The individuality corollary: "persons differ from each other in their construction of events."
- The commonality corollary: "to the extent that one person employs a construction of experience which is similar to that employed by another, his [or her] psychological processes are similar to the other person's."
- The fragmentation corollary: "a person may successively employ a variety of construction subsystems which are infer-

entially incompatible with each other."

· The sociality corollary: "to the extent that one person construes the construction processes of another, he [or she] may play a role in a social process involving the other person."

"On the other hand, Kelly's fundamental view of people as naive scientists was incorporated into most later-developed forms of cognitive-behavioral therapy that blossomed in the late 70s and early 80s and into Intersubjective psychoanalysis which leaned heavily on Kelly's phenomenological perspective and his notion of schematic processing of social information" (Winters, 2013, pp. 276-283). Disordered constructs are those in which the system of construction is not useful in predicting social events and fails to change to accommodate new information. In many ways, Kelly's theory of psychopathology (or mental disorders) is similar to the elements that define a poor theory. A disordered construct system does not accurately predict events or accommodate new data.

You may see that psychodynamic and learning theories differ through time in that the former—Freud et al.— posited drive states that are consistent and become changed when their states are reduced or increased, thereby reinforcing or diminishing learning.

Early behaviorists, like Thorndike and Pavlov, had evidence that learning occurred with brain–environment interactions. Skinner posited operant conditioning, in which the brain had more control over learning than the environment. In the process, he had the individual internalizing its behaviors, again, as in Piaget's child developmental theory.

The cognitive-behavioral psychologists emphasized the *social aspect* of interactions with the environment; then Bandura altered the awareness level in learning theory. Again, he followed the Gestalt tradition of the role of the brain in "representing" the environment, with the brain working from internal maps that allowed the individual to manipulate the environment without participating in it, in short, at a distance.

Internalization led to an individual's "personality" being engaged with social relationships. This furthered the role of personality parameters, enhancing the simpler behaviorist formulation of more rigid brain–environment interactions. You will recall the ancient parallel between "atomism" (behaviorism) and "holism" (analytic–Gestalt) ideas was, and is, still alive and well.

It may thus be clear that, as time and science progress, there is almost never the development of *totally different theories;* rather, there are *alterations of aspects of earlier theories.*

The difference between psychology and non-scientific fields, such as the chemical dependence field based upon the 12- Step Philosophy, is that experiments can be replicated and any changes can be known and measured. If one has only "intuitions" and "hunches," no matter how much inter-rater agreement occurs, this is only a set of assumptions masquerading as "science."

I do not mean to imply that only hard science can be permitted in discussions of human behavior, only that such ideas must be subject to scientific appraisal to be accepted in the larger treatment community.

Prior to such evaluations, these ideas and assumptions can have a heuristic value and allow some practitioners success in treatment and appraisal but not allow the provision of a system of organized teachable and repeatable notions.

If C.D. practitioners always stay within the 12=Step Philosophy and accept its value in dogmatic fashion simply because it has been around a long time, advanced ideas and techniques from scientifically derived parallel fields can be rejected out of hand.

This is a dangerous and self-defeating mind set. Its conservative "purism" becomes only a stodgy and stale approach honoring past founders of a humanistic and caring system.

Humanist Theories

Abraham Maslow

Maslow presented a common-sense idea of a biologically based theory in which the basic physiological needs of humans preceded their psychological needs. He employed a pyramid similar to what the FDA uses for food categories. The bottom of the pyramid had basic survival drives, and the top, self-actualization (Maslow, 1943).

Carl Rogers (1951)

In the mid '50s Rogers moved away from psychoanalysis, which he viewed as more formal and less sensitive to patients' needs in a therapeutic setting.

Person-centered therapy. Rogers originally developed his theory to be the foundation for a system of therapy. He initially called this "non-directive therapy" but later replaced the term "non-directive" with the term "client-centered" and then, later still, used the term "person-centered." Even before the publication of Client-Centered Therapy in 1951, Rogers believed that the principles he was describing could be applied in a variety of contexts and not just in the therapy situation. As a result he started to use the term person-centered approach later in his life to describe his overall theory. Person-centered therapy is the application of the person-centered approach to the therapy situation. Other applications include a theory of personality, interpersonal relations, education, nursing, cross-cultural relations, and other "helping" professions and situations.

The first empirical evidence of the effectiveness of the client-centered approach was published in 1941 at the Ohio State University by Elias Porter using the recordings of therapeutic sessions between Carl Rogers and his clients (Rogers, 1961, p. 84). Porter used Rogers' transcripts to devise a system to measure the degree of directiveness or non-directiveness.

Optimal development, as referred to in proposition 14, results in a certain process rather than static state. He describes this as *the good life*, where the organism continually aims to fulfill its full potential. He listed the characteristics of a fully functioning person (Rogers, 1961):

- A growing openness to experience—they move away from defensiveness and have no need for "subception" (a perceptual defense that involves unconsciously applying strategies to prevent a troubling stimulus from entering consciousness).
- An increasingly existential lifestyle—living each moment fully, not distorting the moment to fit personality or self-concept but allowing personality and self-concept to emanate from the experience. This results in excitement, daring, adaptability, tolerance, spontaneity, and a lack of rigidity, and suggests a foundation of trust. "To open one's spirit to what is going on now, and discover in that present process whatever structure it appears to have."

- Increasing organismic trust, i.e., they trust their own judgment and their ability to choose behavior that is appropriate for each moment. They do not rely on existing codes and social norms but trust that as they are open to experiences they will be able to trust their own sense of right and wrong.

- Freedom of choice—not being shackled by the restrictions that influence an incongruent individual, they are able to make a wider range of choices more fluently. They believe that they play a role in determining their own behavior and so feel responsible for their own behavior.

- Creativity—it follows that they will feel freer to be creative. They will also be more creative in the way they adapt to their own circumstances without feeling a need to conform.

- Reliability and constructiveness—they can be trusted to act constructively. An individual who is open to all their needs will be able to maintain a balance between them. Even aggressive needs will be matched and balanced by intrinsic goodness in congruent individuals.

- A rich, full life—Rogers describes the life of the fully functioning individual as rich, full, and exciting, and suggests that they experience joy and pain, love and heartbreak, fear and courage more intensely. Rogers' description of *the good life*: "This process of the good life is not, I am convinced, a life for the faint-hearted. It involves the stretching and growing of becoming more and more of one's potentialities. It involves the courage to be. It means launching oneself fully into the stream of life" (pp. 84-85).

It is probably clear Rogers' approach is quite different from Freud's and that of others who had highly structured, and perhaps sterile, theories and therapies. His theory and therapy preceded the Existential movement in the U.S. in the 1960s. One of its dominant theorists and therapists was J.F.T. Bugental (1965).

The major thrust of Rogers' approach answered a need for a more humanistic means to establish and maintain a relationship reflected in his theory's name changes: non-directive, client- centered, person-centered. Patients were called "clients," and they felt more involved with their therapists in an emotional and very supportive way.

Neuropsychological/Neurological Theory

Louis Cozolino

Cozolino, a neuropsychologist, helped create the biological therapeutic approach. His theory is based upon the neurological network within the brain and, in that sense, realized Freud's original neurological hope that behavior was brain-based (see Cozolino, 2002):

- "In the future, we may discover scientific evidence that *the interpersonal experience of psychotherapy impacts the neurobiological environment of the brain in ways that stimulate neural plasticity and neurogenesis.*" (p. 39)
- "Emotional factors are more important than the therapist's theoretical orientation." (p. 40)
- "From the perspective of neuroscience, all psychotherapists are in the brain rebuilding business. . . . Repeated attention to

unconscious via confrontation, clarifications, and interpretation results in a gradually expanding awareness on unconscious processes and the integration of top down and left right processing networks" (p. 50). This provides a biological basis for psychoanalysis—Freud's hope."

This is a very important commonality that avoids the frequently ironic notion of different principles among theories that may make no difference in a brain's functioning, or the success we attribute to those specific theories.

 · "Destruction of the amygdala in animals results in an inability to acquire a conditioned fear response. . .the amygdala is well connected, making the fear response a powerful whole body response . . .in the absence of real danger (it) results in panic attacks. (p. 242)

So this changes the historical discussion from trading in behaviors to trading in neuroscience with brain locations and behaviors that may become much more easily and accurately verified.

Psychology as a field only existed as a means of explanation of human behavior, and a very sophisticated one at that. However, from Freud on, many believed the day would come when biology and physical science would supersede it.

One of the interesting outcomes of this line of research and theorizing is that neuroscience has provided evidence, not only for cognitive/behavioral psychology but for all psychologies/psychotherapies. Essentially, it offers a means by which we can measure the efficacy of therapeutic treatments in a far more objective manner.

Chapter Three

PSYCHOTHERAPIES

THOUGH EARLY EXPERIMENTAL/BEHAVIORISTIC theories of human behavior explained how some aspects of our brains worked in normal and educational arenas, there was no focus on neurosis or a therapy. The reason seems to mainly be the result of where each system started—experimental versus clinical settings. So the following will, of course, only discuss clinical therapies from those schools that developed a therapy.

Classical Psychoanalysis

Freud

Psychoanalysis was the first formal psychotherapy in the world. It is possible to view relationships, both personal and professional that employ rapport and transference that lead to comfort and change as therapy does. However, these do not qualify as formal psychotherapy. Further, some therapies did not intend to incorporate these features and yet are under their influence.

Psychoanalysis as developed and employed by Freud set the

structure for other psychoanalytic theories and therapies. This approach, like that of the psychoanalytic theories of others, led to competition; Freud jealously guarded his ideas from change by others, most notably Jung.

It should also be noted that "Freud valued psychoanalysis more as a general theory of civilization than as an individual treatment" (Jacoby, 1983, p. xi).

As the first psychoanalyst, Freud had no one to analyze him. His analysis required him to examine the conscious and unconscious aspects of his life, often enhanced by the thoughts and feelings of his patients—mostly women with hysteria.

Freud's couch was the setting for analysis, and he sat behind his patients. Although this position would perhaps lead us to assume he did so to allow patients to free-associate without his visual interference, he stated otherwise. It was to avoid his seeing patient responses and perhaps responding to them.

Free association, as most people know by now, is the patient's associations as they occur without censorship of content. By doing so, patients begin to experience analytic therapy, which, with dream interpretation, allows an examination of the conscious, pre-conscious, and unconscious areas of the mind.

The overall goal of this therapy is to uncover emotional connections among past associations and to allow emotional, not intellectual, insight to occur. Intellectual insight is relatively useless because it is shallow, without affect, and does not involve lasting change. Additionally, it reinforces obsessional and conscious control over one's life, thereby reducing the actual goal of achieving emotional responses that do lead to change.

This emphasis on emotion, in my opinion, presaged the more recent E.M.D.R. approach that relies on keeping emotion alive in the process of "therapy." However, E.M.D.R. is not a therapy but an adjunct to therapy—more about this later (Shapiro, 2001).

Emotional change, on the other hand, is charged with feeling *of the type that connects with the issue at hand and permits at least partial resolution of that particular issue at that time.* E.M.D.R. requires emotion be present at the same time the threatening picture (target) is kept in mind and kept at as high a level of intensity as possible. Thus, the brief therapist response, "What do you have?"

In my view, there is another aspect of this process that distinguishes most therapies from spontaneous human relationships involving rapport and empathy. It is the manner in which a therapist can share a patient's neurotic experiences via the following metaphor.

In many therapies the therapist, in their mind, observes what is happening from a distance. An example is the patient on a roller coaster and the therapist on the ground. This degree of physical and emotional distance is not as effective an approach as being *in* the roller coaster car with the patient. It is much more real and intense for patient and therapist, as well as more effective.

The initiation of analysis engages the neurosis of the patient with the "transference" process, whereby the patient transfers their neurotic aspects to the analyst. "Counter transference" occurs when the analyst transfers their issues to the patient that interfere with treatment and its primary goal of resolution of the "transference neurosis"—announcing the beginning of the end of treatment.

These processes can occur in all known therapies, whether they are the goal of the therapist or not, and in most other systems they are not. The major problem for non-psychoanalytic therapists is the lack of resolution of these issues, analyzing the transference neurosis as the ending of therapy, because their presence is unknown or unimportant.

When markers are set for change in therapy, they are different in nature from psychoanalysis and more superficial; this difference leads to a different end result.

I was psychoanalyzed at Columbia in the 1960s and became aware of my issues. Once one experiences this, it is not possible to utter glib phrases of assurance about knowing one self, which is common in therapists from some other systems. It is in this regard that Freud stated it is not possible for someone to investigate psychoanalysis without being psychoanalyzed oneself.

With this beginning, he listened very carefully and allowed himself to follow feelings and thoughts with what analyst Theodor Reik said was the "third ear." Reik once interpreted a pregnant patient's dream in which she was in a dentist's chair and had a tooth removed. His next statement was, "Why did you not tell me you had an abortion?" (Reik,1983). Although I do not have the specific page of this remark, it will serve as an example of his thesis that an analyst can employ a greater level of interpretation.

Reik's exchange is typical of an analyst's listening and interpreting, which require knowledge of the treatment approach and one's own psychoanalysis, as well as of one's "observing ego." It is that part of our ego, or self if you will, that allows us to participate and even answer a patient while simultaneously observing ourselves doing so.

This brief introduction to psychoanalysis provides a few techniques that are not present in other treatments. Other approaches to be illustrated later require a face-to-face orientation with straightforward conversation and, of course, awareness of interpretation of thoughts and feelings.

The difference is the depth of interpretation moderated by the therapist's awareness of their own potentially intrusive issues, particularly unconscious ones, and the interference of face-to-face positioning.

Other Psychoanalytic Therapies

These therapies share commonalities with classical psychoanalysis in their reliance on the unconscious with free association and dream interpretation. Beyond this, Horney, for example, emphasized cultural aspects, with women in particular, and discarded Freud's belief in the inherited/instinctual superiority of men.

Her therapy would permit women and men to expect change to come more easily since it is not a "given" and could involve a change in perception and programming.

"The goal of therapy for Horney is to help people resolve their defenses that alienate them from their true likes and dislikes, hopes, fears, and desires—so that they can get in touch with what she called their 'real selves'." (Paris, 1998, p. 238).

Erik Erikson

Horney's system of ideas was quite sophisticated and well developed as a representative of the Neo-Freudian School. A later development occurred with Erik Erikson. As noted earlier, he was an admirer of Freud and provided a theory, and later a therapy, derived from it that conserved the classical theory's valuable ideas and practices while advancing the social dimension of the Neo-Freudians, though not necessarily in a manner they would have necessarily agreed with.

The chart shown earlier provides parallel stages between Freud and Erikson. Though Erikson did not personally develop Ego-Psychoanalytic Psychotherapy, the system was broader than the classical psychoanalytic one.

It emphasized the patient's life outside the treatment hour in a different way. For example, a patient may have phallic issues—sex organ involvement that presages adoption of adult sexual behavior. The added social dimension involved the child's, and now adult's, initiative in moving forward with such behaviors, but also has its opposite, a sense of guilt about not following parental prohibitions.

A famous dictum of Erikson's was, "The child is father to the man." This represented the idea that adults, no matter how old, still have childhood experiences and unresolved stages that control their lives. So, regardless of the theory or therapy that maintains otherwise, the long past matters, and we and our patients disregard it at our peril in avoiding the completeness necessary for a balanced therapeutic outcome and life. Another contribution of Erikson's is his notion of triple bookkeeping—that understanding a person requires taking into account somatic factors, social context, and ego development—all in relation to each other (Erikson, 1953).

I recall an actual example from the old T.C. model, specifically at Liberty Village, in which a bed-wetting resident was provided with the depression-era "sandwich board" posters that, in his case, said, *I'm a baby, treat me like one.* To enhance the embarrassment further, he was given an infant's hat, clothes, and a baby bottle.

I had the responsibility of resolving this and proceeded in a different manner. His nocturnal enuresis was a probable inherited behavior with a regressive response to stress in his life and inpatient existence, *not* a behavior he could control.

By deciding it was controllable, the residential recovering staff placed responsibility on him and further stressed him so the behavior and his development was unwittingly protracted—not the goal the staff and resident desired.

My solution was to treat the problem with a behaviorist technique. Sears sold a device based upon Mowrer's psychological theory. It was comprised of two sheets of aluminum connected at their ends and attached to a battery and bell. Bed sheets were placed between the aluminum "sheets" to prevent the bell going off until both sheets were wet from urine.

During the night, he would void and the bell would go off. That awoke him, of course, and he arose, showered, changed his pajamas, cleaned the bed, replaced the sheets, and then fell asleep again.

This was repeated for about ten days, when the bedwetting ended—miraculously—in the staff's view. The SR connection was a bell to disrupt his sleep and make him more sensitive to his body's signal to void, which he then responded to in a normal manner.

The process allowed him to avoid the pain of embarrassment and the futility of the TC "treatment." More importantly, it was one of several instances that allowed the staff to be exposed to alternate, more sophisticated and scientific, techniques they were unaware of. They were not mental health professionals—just recovering people.

The end result was their growing confidence in my "magic" that permitted them to refer problem residents. We then had conversations in treatment committees, which I set up as clinical director, to begin the change in modality. I should mention, my strong relationship with the staff was significantly enhanced by my knowledge of a recovering staff member I knew from our area of residence. These serendipitous occurrences move activities in directions not likely to happen without them.

To continue with our theoretical discussion, another addition was Erikson's theoretical stages into old age. This moved the change issues and opportunities from that ending with adolescence and applied them into the entire life span. Older adult stages present their somewhat different problems and resolutions.

Along with the therapeutic difference, analytic hours were less frequent, three times/week instead of five or more, more broadly enlarging the scope of response. It focused on more real-life behaviors and emphasized the environmental influences, deemphasizing inherited behaviors, which were still there and regarded as such. In this respect, Psychoanalysis moved closer to Cognitivism.

Behaviorist Theories

B.F. Skinner

Although there are behaviorist theories applied to therapies, there is not now in general practice a "Behavioral Therapy" but rather a combined "Cognitive Behavioral Therapy" with the emphasis on cognition. More relevantly, there is no "Skinnerian Therapy" as far as I know. There is the practice of Skinner's principles to educational settings—with rats in mazes and students in classrooms. The key factor here is the clean application of simple, cogent principles to simple behaviors

Exposure Therapies–PTSD

Reciprocal Inhibition (Joseph Wolpe)

Wolpe developed "Reciprocal Inhibition"—a process of relearning whereby in the presence of a stimulus, a non-anxiety-producing response, is continually repeated until it is extinguishes the old, undesirable response. This is "a variety of the techniques based on reciprocal inhibition, such as systematic desensitization, avoidance conditioning, and the use of assertion" (Wolpe et al., 1958, p. 114).

A practical example of R.I. would be a patient fearful of height who is asked about their levels of fear at various heights and places. The examples are then placed on a spectrum of least-to-most anxiety-producing examples.

Then the least fearful stimuli—using a ladder to paint a ceiling for example—are thought about at the same time and are paired with non-threatening stimuli, such as a relaxing scene. The continual representation of such stimuli will diminish the higher heights, thereby hopefully ending or diminishing the person's fear.

Implosion

Implosive Therapy is based on the principle of exposing the patient to trauma-related cues until there is a reduction in anxiety associated with the cues.

PTSD

By remaining relaxed as successive cues are presented, the patient learns to associate the cues with feelings of relaxation rather than with anxiety.

Flooding

"Implosive Therapy" involves only imagining stimuli (without direct contact). In Flooding, the patient is relaxed and then presented with a "flood" of their most feared traumatic experience, which allows the anxiety to diminish, respectively, helpful in treating combat veterans with PTSD.

Stress Inoculation Training (SIT)

Stress Inoculation Training (SIT) is a skills-focused anxiety management approach that includes relaxation training, social skills, and distraction techniques. All three methodologies are similar, in that fear is at the base of PTSD.

Although this set of approaches is clearly more effective than psychoanalysis, as Wolpe states, its relatively simple action is also clearly very important to a suffering patient. The major point is that behavioristic and cognitive approaches in theory and therapy have, over time, collapsed examples of human suffering into much smaller categories that are easier to deal with.

Whether this was planned or shifted to satisfy thinking at the time, *it had the effect of making the experiments and applications easier to resolve and to measure.* This idea will be presented repeatedly because it characterizes the major restructuring of the analytic versus cognitive/behavioral views of scientific research and therapy.

No matter how admirable, this approach is very different from making a much larger theory verifiable and at the same time tackling the issues of, e.g., guilt, morality, and anomie—none of which diminishes the value of this superior therapeutic approach in the resolution of smaller issues, only that it places its value within a historical therapeutic context that has, over time, changed the direction of psychological thinking.

E.M.D.R.

Eye Movement Desensitization and Reprocessing (E.M.D.R.) was developed by Francine Shapiro (1995).

The incident that led to this discovery was a walk in a park in New York City. She thought of a traumatic event in her life that, she believed, led to her eyes making peculiar movements. When she verified this later with her colleagues, she theorized that, if the thought led to the eye movements, then eye movements could possibly lead to resolution of the trauma.

When a person experiences a traumatic event—rape, or a war incident, for example—a dysfunctional response can occur. The person becomes intensely upset, and their heart rate, breathing, and blood pressure increase. The person then attempts to convince their mind that the re-experienced event is not real, so they can slow down the process to a more relaxed state.

As a short term "fix," it seems to work. However, this process, called a "closed-loop behavior," recurs again and again without change, harassing the individual ad infinitum.

The early E.M.D.R. attempts to elicit trauma resolution involved horizontal hand movements by the therapist while the patient recalled a picture of the trauma and the emotional state at this time, followed by its location in their body, then their assessment of the severity of the feeling state on a 0–10 scale called the S.U.D. (Subjective Unit of Disturbance) with 0 representing "nothing at all" and 10 a "maximum disturbance."

It is notable that authors who may not be aware of the changes in procedure typically mention the horizontal hand movements only, as though no other improvements have occurred since its initiation. Although, while in training, we were taught to use our fingers in a horizontal manner to mimic the early work, I know of no certified E.M.D.R. therapist who uses their fingers instead of a device. It is also recommended that you ask the therapist whether they are "certified" and have a certificate.

The earliest device (EYE SCAN—NeuroTek Corp.com.) to go beyond therapists' hand movements was a long bar on a tripod with horizontally moving lights accompanied with pulsars—pulsating vibrators held in the hands—and a headset that produced alternating beeps in each ear.

The lights, pulses, and beeps all alternate left–right together. The purpose of this arrangement is to disrupt the brain's dysfunctional attempts to deal with the trauma in closed-loop behavior fashion. The latest device, in 1990, was a single unit and was called the LapScan—later, LapScan 4000. It looks like a small blackboard in a wooden frame with lights and outlets for beeps and pulsars (vibrating pads).

The assumption has been that trauma occurs and is stored in STM instead of LTM, where it is more closely aligned with consciousness and its ability to interfere with one's functioning. Some believe this storage location is the wrong place; others, like me, believe it is Nature's way of providing an immediate reminder for the person to not repeat the traumatic event.

E.M.D.R. differs from other approaches above in not requiring any real-life stimuli that may be too threatening for the person. It is employed for all sorts of trauma, e.g., war trauma, and is recommended by the Department of Defense (DOD) for returning soldiers)—see emdr.com. It is useful for all sorts of trauma resolution as well, like rape, bullying, phobias, etc.

There is a process (Shapiro, 1995, p. 67) of preparation the first time to familiarize the patient with the entire procedure before any therapeutic work is begun. The next step is to establish "targets" by taking a history of events and ranking them accordingly with regard to intensity, *as the patient sees them.*

The patient is then asked to recall the target event with its accompanying affect, which is amplified as much as possible by the therapist to lead to as much resolution as possible. It is most important to restate, as in other approaches, the initial target(s) are not the *most* intense, but *lesser* intense ones. The event, with accompanying affect, body location, and intensity, are then restated by the therapist just before the device is turned on.

The stimuli from the device are initiated, and the therapist decides how long the cycle will continue. On average it probably runs for 1–2 minutes, depending on patient responses and the therapist's assessment of the situation. It is not the goal to make the patient as comfortable as possible, nor is it to make the patient unduly uncomfortable, only emotionally aware and pressured.

To explain further, the goal is to allow the brain to re-experience the trauma in face of the emotional response, which essentially convinces the brain it can survive, adjust to the trauma, and in the process reduce ("desensitize") and relax to the point of resolution ("reprocess").

Subsequent to the desensitizing and reprocessing, the mind

shifts to clearer thinking and begins to resolve the issue with rational views and steps to make life more comfortable and more under the subject's control.

During re-presenting of the trauma event again and again, it is important for the therapist not to stop after each cycle and begin a therapeutic conversation. To do so would reduce the intensity of the affect state and thereby movement toward resolution. The measure of resolution of *that particular event* is the decreasing of the SUD score from some higher score to as close as possible to "0". It is assumed that reaching close to "0" is the point of resolution, and the hoped-for end of trauma-related symptoms, as it moves from STM to LTM. Typically, as the intensity level drops, the patient becomes a bit more tired, and some patients even ask to move on to another target or to stop.

The next step is to move to another target decided upon by patient and therapist. The target's relationships begin to resemble a road map of sorts—with a "town" being resolved and then perhaps the choosing of another "town" nearby. At some further point the patient begins to feel more comfortable with the process and its conflict resolution.

There are other approaches besides resolution of past events, and one is called a "future template." This involves an event that has not yet occurred and can be targeted and reduced in anxiety level before it happens. Examples of this are very important job interviews, exams, promotion discussions, etc.

A comparison of E.M.D.R. with some more involved therapeutic enterprise like psychoanalysis makes them seem farther apart than they might be, with the former as a "cognitive" approach and the latter as an "analytic" one. However, E.M.D.R. is not terribly cognitive, with its ability to arouse significant affect and elicit unconscious information.

My metaphor, which allows a comparison with other therapies, is that of an accordion or concertina with ribs in its flexible and moving bellows. When the bellows are expanded, the ribs are farthest apart, and if we represent the ribs as insight events in an analytic approach, they occur at infrequent and distant points. Conversely, when the bellows are closed, the ribs are closer together and represent the insight opportunities as more frequent, such as occurs with E.M.D.R.

Since the E.M.D.R. approach provides this, the therapist has an easier job of making emotionally insightful connections. If we recall, earlier cognitive behavioral therapies did not involve emotional insight as a *formal* part of their resolution—E.M.D.R. and some other treatments require it.

In this respect, E.M.D.R. is "accelerated" analysis, in my opinion. An additional point—E.M.D.R. allows a therapist with average ability to perform at a more effective therapeutic level by reaching deeper issues sooner.

In my practice I have joined E.M.D.R. with an analytic or cognitive approach to initiate quicker and more effective progress. The initial seating arrangement is face-to-face conversation in sessions, with early decisions about whether we first choose some type of therapy or E.M.D.R. Sometimes sessions are all talk, sometimes all E.M.D.R., and sometimes both.

As an example, a patient may wish to choose to talk only, but as we progress, a target may present itself, and they, or I, might suggest we try E.M.D.R. In this way the patient is in shared control of the session and is thus more active and invested in its progress.

I have added the use of complimentary relaxation CDs to this approach to allow patients to practice at home, between sessions. One CD is a direct recording of the headphones' "beeps"—30 minutes' worth. This has been most helpful when used for clearing a busy mind—one full of racing or random thoughts—with the statement to "let it go," said to oneself, to empty the mind.

It is valuable for some practitioners to decide whether the basis for this symptom is ADD or a mood state that would be better dealt with first by medication. If the practitioner and patient resist the idea of medication, then of course they should consider proceeding without them.

The second CD is what I call "Color Relaxation," as taught by my E.M.D.R trainer. It involves a patient picturing a colored ball (with a color the patient finds relaxing), perhaps the size of a soccer ball on top of their head, with the color then transferring itself, first to their brain cavity, then downward through their body's major organs and muscles, and out through the toes.

The key aspect is to speak slowly and in a low, relaxed voice, with distinct spaces between words and sentences. When you have made your way to and out of the toes, you can instruct the patient to: (a) "think of something positive you truly believe about yourself, and only when you are ready, open your eyes," or alternately, (b) instead of opening their eyes, they can just lie there and rest, or allow themselves to fall asleep. It is important that the CDs are used at home in a supine position, with legs and arms uncrossed.

This combination of therapies and CDs provides patients with the best chance to progress, and they are also more likely to be committed to therapy. I will provide a more comparative discussion in the final chapter among all theories and therapies, but so far you may see how we can join effective therapies to achieve greater progress.

Therapeutic examples. This female patient, L, was forty-seven years old at the time, and is the eldest of three children, with a sister three years her junior and a brother nine years her junior. We had employed earlier, less intense targets before her wanting to pursue one involving herself, her siblings, and her father, who had been a policeman in their youth.

Before she was referred to me, she had been diagnosed as a manic-depressive, with appropriate meds for that condition and a social worker providing psychotherapy. My evaluation did not confirm the diagnosis, because there was no mania—only psychotic thoughts and behavior that required quarterly hospitalizations for one month each, taking this amount of time from her schedule as a teacher. She looked forward to the quiet withdrawal from her life as the time for inpatient hospitalizations approached.

The psychiatrist I chose confirmed her diagnosis as Major Depression Recurrent with psychotic features and changed her medications. This led to markedly improved functioning and no further inpatient treatment except for one, when she was diagnosed with cancer that threatened her life. I had had her in treatment for five years at that point and did not try E.M.D.R. until long after she became non-psychotic.

The target involved her youthful recall of her father aggressively telling the three children where he would be storing his weapon, on top of the refrigerator. She thought this was dangerous and absurd, and cursed his behavior for scaring them, but especially her younger brother, who was fearful of him for decades afterwards.

The initial target (the picture) was his speaking to them as he put the gun on the refrigerator, saying, " I don't want any of you #%&! kids touching this." Her feelings were: rage, fear, and disgust. Location in her body: stomach, chest and throat, SUD-10.

After running the lights and pulsars for about two minutes, I stopped and asked, "What do you have?" (Not a therapeutic, "How do you feel?" or "Tell me more.") "Deep breath in and out"; she delayed her response and expressed an uncharacteristic level of anger. She said, "How could he do this? Didn't he realize how dangerous and scary this was? (SUD?) "Still 10"

Cycle—end— (Continue with where you left off.) — Stop— "I am still angry." (Did anything change?) I am trying to see how it was from his point of view, because my parents are good people and they must have meant well, but this was stupid!"

Cycle—end— ("What do you have?") "I am not as angry—he did something very bad, but I see why he wanted us to be afraid so as not to ever touch it." ("Is anything else changing?") "Yes, I went somewhere else to other things he did that were kinder" SUD-6.

Note her level of anger dropping while her mind focuses on

"other things"—this occurs when the affect of the initial target is lowering in value. It is a harbinger of what is to come—resolution of this issue. Her affect is quieter also, with less intensity.

> Cycle—end— *"I'm trying to regain my anger, but it is slipping away. I'm coming to terms with my anger and his behavior. I identify with his actions because I'm a parent and I could respond like him in the right circumstances"* SUD-3-4.
>
> Cycle—end— *"I'm becoming disinterested in this, starting to feel tired, but I don't know why."* *("One more trial, please.")*
>
> Cycle—end— *"Now I am tired. Could we stop?"* *("Tell me what occurred,")* and the SUD score is near zero. *"I can't get upset, and I'm okay with it now; I can't keep this trauma in my mind forever."*

The end is clear with her affect and thoughts running dry. At this point the issue seems resolved, and the target is presumed to have moved from STM to LTM, where we want it to be.

Should this have arisen again, we would have reengaged the target and dropped the SUD value further, or back to zero if it increased. In reality, this never reemerged. The entire set of cycles lasted about twenty-five minutes, which was fairly typical and rapid. Compare this with the amount of time and effort to use another standard therapeutic system.

Patients J & G-Pain Relief. I have two patients with neurocognitive issues: One has Post-Concussive Disorder, and the other primarily Dementia.

The Post-Concussive Disorder patient, J, is now forty-six and was a passenger in a car that was hit from the front and back, forcing him through the windshield. He remembers nothing from the moment of the crash except that he believes he clicked on his seat belt.

His symptoms included cognitive confusion, headaches and backaches, and memory loss; he immediately forgot phone conversations with his clients just after he hung up. He had great limitations with deductive reasoning examples, such as those given by his cognitive therapist. He also had blurry vision that led to dizziness and nausea, then to emesis.

He had great difficulty walking and required a walker and cane. He cannot drive a car and is not permitted to do so. He is not able to perform his job as an insurance broker and works from his home with extensive help from his office assistant.

I should mention his disabilities are so great that he must be seen at home; before the accident, he was seen in my New York City office.

Prior to the accident in March 2014, he was a very effective agent working from early morning to late evening, and dating women on evenings and weekends. Now he is house bound, and when I first met him he was only capable of working ten to fifteen minutes a day, with pain and confusion that ended his continuance. He had difficulty getting out of bed and fell several times, resulting in further head injury.

I had seen him as an office patient years earlier and provided therapy and, later, E.M.D.R. for his anxiety and OCD style of functioning. So he was comfortable with the E.M.D.R. process, and this made resuming therapy easy.

I offered to use E.M.D.R. to relax him and perhaps provide some hope for the future. He had a very fatalistic view of what the future held and said many times, "I'm never going to be the same as I was, and things will get worse." My plan was to do what I could to relieve his hopelessness.

We started the E.M.D.R. process, which was of course not as effective as his pre-accident functioning. I noticed as we proceeded that the lights were a major problem. I had checked earlier with his neurologist for permission to use lights, since he might have had seizures or the propensity for them. The neurologist had said there was no risk with lights, but they bothered him, so I stopped them.

I then employed headphones and pulsars, and they worked better. Specifically, I noted his mental confusion sometimes interfered with progress, and I then employed only the headphone beeps. This works well with any patients who have busy, overly full minds.

The beeps, with directions to focus on them, allow patients to let go of busy thoughts, and this works very well in all circumstances in which I've used it, and did with him as well.

We noted the beeps cleared his mind well enough to increase his effective work time from ten to fifteen minutes per day to two to three hours! We both found this surprising and very welcome, because he began to be less fatalistic about his future. My initial plan to only decrease his anxiety had apparently been too modest.

He still had head and back pain on a regular basis, which led me to try the pulsars as a solution. These were administered while he lay down to relieve the stress on his back. The back pain in this instance occurred a few days after he received a strong epidural type medicine and was accompanied by a headache, which he thought would interfere with us doing any work.

We proceeded, and I allowed fifteen minutes for the process to continue without interruption from me. When I stopped the pulsar vibrations and asked him how he felt, he said the pain was mostly gone. My assumption is the stimulus had acted as a distraction so his brain would not focus on the pain. I was very surprised that both these approaches worked in ways I had never thought possible.

After this success, I mentioned that an objective test would be his engaging the beeps prior to a session with his cognitive therapist to see if there was any improvement at their session.

An important challenge was two deductive reasoning examples she used—which he could never solve, even after many months of presentation. He not only solved them both, but told his therapist there were two possible solutions to one of the problems!

Besides cognitive therapy, he had weekly sessions for physical therapy, vestibular treatment and, as needed, neurological checks, psychiatric medication checks, and C-PAP machine adjustments. In spite of all of these approaches, nothing had led to any improvement, except truncated E.M.D.R. and recent back surgery to cauterize nerves and reduce pain.

I have searched for articles on E.M.D.R. being used in this way and could find nothing similar; effectiveness of the On-The-Spot Method (Amana & Toichi, 2014, pp. 50-65). The authors shorten the Eight-Step E.M.D.R. process due to limitations of dementia patients and employ only tapping—alternately touching the patient's knees with the therapist's fingers.

In subsequent sessions, this patient proceeded to make progress with his symptomatology. An old dream was discussed in which he became paralyzed and woke, unable to move. This of course frightened him, and he would not permit himself to sleep in the daytime when his female partner was not around. At night, she could help him wake up and move.

The dream consisted of his being a passenger in a car with other people he did not know, all of whom are in shadow, and one man with a hood who laughed at him derisively.

We began E.M.D.R. with this target, accompanying emotions and location in the body and an SUD score of 10. In the recall portion, he said the man appeared to be evil and this led to great anxiety. I viewed his issues from an analytic perspective, though I was employing a non-analytic therapeutic approach.

I suggested he change the target and view the man as a person who is giving feedback about his present and future perspective; this led to a much different response—more relaxed and clearer in meaning.

Prior to this outcome, he asked about a medicine for his PTSD dream, and I checked with a psychiatrist who recommended Mini-Press, which is specific for such issues.

He then spoke about his pre-accident womanizing and high living which, in turn, had led to his seeing the figure as helpful and as himself, and about how the figure was laughing at his foolishness and mistakes made. However, the accident led to his meeting a woman who genuinely loves him, with a child from a previous man. He regards this as a "gift." This E.M.D.R. session led to ongoing relief from symptoms, and the Mini-Press may be unnecessary at some future time.

In subsequent months to the present, when the book is finished, he had improved pain relief from what we first employed. However, he had cervical disc deterioration in seven to eight discs, and the surgeon chose three vertebrae to operate upon.

Titanium metal attached with some rotational R.O.M. (Range Of Motion) limitation, but pain relief has been significant, and he can walk without a cane or walker for periods and in a clear vertical position. At the time of publication, he has much less pain and is looking forward to more back surgery.

Additional work involved RehaCom (2016), a software program that essentially retrains the brain to perform tasks it could not previously. In several sessions, he was able to make remarkable improvement in memory, which is his greatest weakness.

I am entering my final note about his progress just before publication. Rehacom has improved his memory better than any other approach. He made another observation, that Rehacom allowed him to return to thinking on "multi-levels" at one time.

For example, prior to the accident he was able to think of many different issues, clients, etc., and keep track of them. He is not able to do this quite yet, but he can handle some tasks which he has only been able to do since Rehacom training.

I don't have research evidence to document this, but it appears Rehacom trains the mind to do related aspects of whatever the main training task is—in this case, memory function. He is happier and more hopeful than at anytime since I began working with him, and he now believes because of his progress he could be employable someday. Once again, Rehacom does more than I expected!

The second patient, G., is a physician, sixty-three years of age and a runner. While running in a foreign country, he fell on an unfinished road with large gravel and fractured his jaw. Subsequent to this, his memory faltered badly, and he forgot simple things like his keys, phone, and pen. He also forgot names of common things and people he knew. When speaking, he would stumble on words or forget them altogether.

His high-level position at a medical school was taken from him, and he could no longer see hospital patients—a devastating blow that suggested the end of his career, and psychic death in his view as well.

His evaluating physicians found no positive data from gross neurological, CAT, and MRI scans. I administered a neuropsychological test (R.B.A.N.S.) and verified the severe loss of types of memory and gross eye–hand coordination tasks.

I suggested that the extended series of evaluations with onerous implications were too stressful, and that E.M.D.R. should be employed to relieve his anxiety and hopelessness. He had difficulty with the standard E.M.D.R. procedure—establishing and maintaining the target, and holding the emotional connection with the target "picture."

He tried to cooperate but could not and sometimes seemed frustrated. I switched away from the standard procedure and provided him with two CDs—beeps, and color relaxation.

The most effective procedure was an older format from Herbert Spencer (1975), who developed a "Calm Scene." This procedure involved his finding the image of the calmest scene from a place the patient had actually been.

In his case it was not a place in the usual sense—sunny beach, country place, a special room. Since he was a runner, that activity was calming and led to the most relaxing state he could think of, as well as one that surprised him and me. As a psychiatrist and neurologist, when he thought of running, his body reacted, not only in his mind, but in his arms and legs, since nerves and muscles contracted as though he were actually running.

The relaxed state mimicked the standard E.M.D.R. procedure in its effect. He was relatively anxiety-free, and we could continue with a standard therapy approach. It allowed him to focus and empathize with himself and others, as well as to consider the possibility of his serious diagnosis. This set of thoughts was in his preconscious and occasionally protruded, sometimes in angry fashion.

Other improvements included less forgetfulness and a smoother relationship with his life. His response to the procedures was presumably the same as those of patient number one in that distraction worked. However, of course, no procedures of this kind could reverse his neurocognitive changes.

Is Distraction the Basis for This Phenomenon?

"'Diffuse noxious inhibitory controls' (DNIC), a form of supraspinal descending endogenous analgesia, requires a noxious conditioning stimulus for pain attenuation. This may be partly dependent on a distraction effect. The term 'conditioned pain modulation' (CPM) has recently been introduced to describe the psychophysical paradigm to test DNIC. The present study aimed to determine whether distraction and tonic heat stimulation inhibit pain through the same or different mechanisms by looking at whether there is a similar or even an additive effect on pain attenuation. Test pain was brief heat stimulation applied to the left volar of 34 healthy volunteers. For conditioning, the right hand was immersed in 46.5° C water. Distraction was provided by three different difficulty levels of continuous cognitive visual tasks. Experimental blocks consisted of test pain: (1) alone; *'baseline'*, (2) with conditioning pain; 'CPM', (3) with distraction; *'distraction'* and (4) with conditioning pain and distraction; *'combined'*. They were randomized and repeated three times and pain intensity and unpleasantness rated. Results showed an overall effect of experimental block on test pain intensity ($P = 0.0125$). Post-hoc tests revealed a significant reduction in pain intensity ratings under Combined (21.2 ± 2.3; mean $\pm$ SEM) compared to CPM alone (16.0 ± 2.3) ($P < 0.05$). Furthermore, at all levels of distraction there were always a few subjects who were not distracted despite expressing CPM. Based on the additive effect of CPM and distraction on pain inhibition, and the cases of no distraction despite CPM, we suggest that CPM acts independently from distraction" (Moont, Pud, Sprecher, Sarvit, & Yarnitsky, 2010, pp. 113-120).

Alfred A. Borrelli

Chapter Four

EVALUATING CLINICAL COMPARISONS OF DIFFERING MENTAL HEALTH PROFESSIONALS' SKILL LEVELS

Counseling and Psychotherapy

AS A FOREWORD TO THIS SECTION, I would suggest the reader not view this exposition of theories as more than informative, and not "choose sides" according to what your brain's orientation or past experience and training tell you. Allow yourself to read these words without prejudice, and even consider how ideas from a "foreign" field might be acceptable and worked into the field you already know.

Counseling is usually regarded as a means of treating someone by employing conscious, here-and-now, straightforward discussions with clients that allow them to understand the conundrums of their behaviors and choose ways to end the conflicts and queries.

It almost always involves face-to-face approaches and even completions of surveys, diaries (journals), and writing letters to others who are part of their conflicts. The goal of counseling is to permanently resolve issues, but amelioration of symptoms is an adequate end game.

Psychotherapy is more varied and complex. Essentially, it includes a spectrum of approaches from conscious to unconscious modes, and from face-to-face to couch work, in which the patient often has no eye contact with the therapist.

The goal of either approach is to achieve permanent behavior change. The personality theories supporting these therapies are more complex as well, ranging from behavioristic through cognitive to analytic ones, with variations of all, and new ones besides, as we have already seen.

Nominal, Ordinal, Interval, and Ratio Scales

Many statistics books begin by defining the different kinds of variables you might wish to analyze. This system was developed by Stevens (1951, pp. 1-49):

"A *categorical* variable, also called a *nominal* variable, is for mutual exclusive, but not ordered, categories. For example, your study might compare five different genotypes. You can code the five genotypes with numbers if you want, but the order is arbitrary and any calculations (for example, computing an average) would be meaningless.

"An *ordinal* variable is one where the order matters but not the difference between values. For example, you might ask patients to express the amount of pain they are feeling on a scale of 1 to 10. A score of 7 means more pain than a score of 5, and that is more than a score of 3. But the difference between the 7 and the 5 may not be the same as that between 5 and 3. The values simply express an order.

"The difference between a temperature of 100 degrees and 90 degrees is the same difference as between 90 degrees and 80 degrees. A *ratio* variable, has all the properties of an interval variable, and also has a clear definition of 0.0.'no heat'.

"Another counter example is PH. It is not a ratio variable, as pH=0 just means 1 molar of H+, and the definition of molar is fairly arbitrary. A pH of 0.0 does not mean 'no acidity' (quite the opposite!). When working with ratio variables, but not interval variables, you can look at the ratio of two measurements.

"A weight of 4 grams is twice a weight of 2 grams, because weight is a ratio variable. A temperature of 100 degrees C is not twice as hot as 50 degrees C, because temperature C is not a ratio variable. A pH of 3 is not twice as acidic as a pH of 6, because pH is not a ratio variable."

Such use of categorization has worked well for many years. However, in this section my approach will focus, not on comparisons of techniques, but on comparisons of professionals who make judgments employing these techniques. Psychiatrists employ DSM-V. The technique employed, like all techniques, controls what practitioners see.

Since the DSM names things in its categorization, syndromes in this case—it does little more, and that keeps it at a *nominal* level. So, any questions about diagnoses at a higher level would be difficult to derive

The scales above (Stevens, 1946, pp. 677-680) indicate a spectrum of measures/tests developed to assess the relative sophistication of DSM diagnoses. My approach is to compare and contrast these as the DSM-V for psychiatrists—as well as practitioners' use of this categorization scheme.

Besides this academically derived mnemonic's use for categorization, I wish to draw broader attention to the manner in which our use of any system not only aids organization but, more importantly, narrows our view of adopting other systems and being objective about the system we are using. *In this respect, the system can control us.*

So we might rate the four types of mental health practitioners— counselors, social workers, psychologists, and psychiatrists. All are capable, of course, but some are more capable than others—types and individuals—in terms of evaluating mental health dysfunction, in this case.

The issues of accuracy and objectivity are relevant here. If a counselor employs a test, the vast majority of which have been developed by psychologists, it is a more objective and accurate approach.

However, if a psychiatrist were to employ the DSM in a verbal setting *with no tests*, he or she is not employing a more objective approach but may be *more accurate in the assessment* compared to the counselor/psychologist *with* tests. The difference lies in skill and experience. However, if we were to control for skill and experience, tests would carry the day.

Psychiatry-Genomind

The DSM has had its problems since its inception in 1952 and one of its current major critics is Allen Frances (2013, pp. 128-129), an American psychiatrist best known for chairing the task force that produced the fourth revision of *Diagnostic and Statistical Manual,* DSM-IV-TR, and for his critique of the current version, DSM-5. I have quoted liberally from this publication, since he speaks in a very pithy manner.

He warns that the expanding boundary of psychiatry is causing a diagnostic inflation that is swallowing up normality, and that the over-treatment of the "worried well" is distracting attention from the core mission of treating the more severely ill. In 2013, Frances (p. 128) said, "Psychiatric diagnosis still relies exclusively on fallible subjective judgments rather than objective biological tests."

DSM

"Despite its conservative intent and careful methodology, DSM-IV was not able to prevent diagnostic inflation. Rates of attention deficit disorder tripled as a result of heavy drug company marketing starting in 1997—instigated by the introduction of new on-patent drugs and facilitated by the removal of federal prohibitions against direct-to-consumer advertising. Rates of autism increased by more than twentyfold, largely because the loose diagnosis followed it's becoming a prerequisite for extra school services. Rates of bipolar disorder doubled largely because of drug company marketing. And rates of bipolar disorder in children increased by fortyfold when thought-leaders and drug companies convinced practitioners that temperamental kids had bipolar disorder even if they didn't have mood swings—a concept that had been rejected by DSM-IV." Frances later felt that DSM-IV should have fought more vigorously against the risks of diagnostic inflation by tightening diagnostic criteria and providing more specific warnings against over-diagnosis. Frances co-authored *Am I Okay? A Layman's Guide to the Psychiatrist's Bible* (2000).

"Most who oppose DSM-V do not reject the classification of mental disorders. We consider it essential for epidemiology, research, and clinical work. What we *do* contest is the specific reliability, validity, and usefulness [of] new DSM-V diagnoses and also the closed and disorganized way in which it was prepared" (Frances, 2013, pp. 128-129).

These direct quotes should make it widely clear the DSM has been a compilation of verbal statements, which have been vague on occasion, and had had its labeling directed by major drug companies to promote their medications, as well by as insurance companies that desired more accurate information.

In recent years insurance companies have moved toward biological, genetic labels which note that such syndromes, being biologically based, could be viewed in the same way as medical treatment and, therefore, had no automatic time/session limitation. This mimics the long-standing rules already in existence for MDs in their treatment of patients.

As a corollary, psychiatric syndromes such as manic depression, severe depression, and obsessive-compulsive disorder, considered bio-based, are treated within this same framework.

Of course, one glaring omission is ADD (ADHD), which is clearly inherited and therefore biologically based. I suspect insurance companies do not wish to open this Pandora's box to a vast number of people with varying degrees of debilitation.

Dr. Frances's desire that DSMs should be more biologically

based with evidence is laudable (see GENOMIND). This clearly has been the goal of medical assessment in all areas since Freud, and while we don't have the scientific evidence to do a lot, we can begin the search.

Louis Cozolino's (2002) ideas in *The Neuroscience of Psychotherapy* will be presented later and provide a biological basis for some of Frances's ideas about refining the DSM versions in a more accurate and physiological fashion.

The DSM has begun the classification by naming different syndromes with different symptoms, requiring different verbal and medication treatments.

Nominal, Ordinal, Interval, and Ratio Scales, and Their Implications for Mental Health Practitioners and the DSM

As noted earlier, "Statistical data in psychology have four types: nominal, ordinal, interval and ratio. Nominal consists of named categories such as male or female. Ordinal allows classification such as greater than or less than. Interval compares items that are measured in equal distances, such as inches or feet. Ratio refers to interval data that have a known starting point. Data types are important because they determine which, if any, statistical tests are appropriate in their analysis" (Stevens, 1946, pp. 677-680).

Although these authors are correct, in my view, besides types of statistical treatments, the categories can also come to represent the process of rational thinking by mental health practitioners. In other words, broadly speaking, practitioners think and have thought in terms of these four types of statistical treatments. I am saying that those who employ a naming system like the DSM are limiting their purview to only that system's basic level of analysis.

This issue is common to all systems of classification, not just the DSM, of course; but there is always a need to use a more variegated and sophisticated system. Frances argues for a biologically based system that moves us in that direction. However, biology is not the only approach to be considered, and it may be premature at this stage of the field's development. Factor analysis, a statistical treatment, is probably more valuable at present.

This brings us to psychological statistics. The application to the DSM would be as follows. If the problem with the DSM is its nominal quality—just names for syndromes—then it needs to move to the ordinal level at least, to increase its sophistication. That level measures "more than or less than." With factor analysis it might then *be* at the ordinal level—*and* with improved relationships among syndromes, since that is what factor analysis provides.

Regarding a nominal classification, in DSM terms, can we say that one syndrome is more or less than another? Is schizophrenia more or less than manic depression? Are both of these more or less than dysthymia? *These judgments are qualitative, not quantitative,* and as such, by definition preclude quantification.

Before proceeding to other mental health fields' systems levels, we might explain that the *nominal-to-ratio scheme* is not just a system designed to allow different statistical treatments to be applied. As I have already noted, the clinical systems employed limit the practitioners' views while they attempt to broaden it—more names, but only at the same level of description/accuracy that guides their interpretations.

For example, if the DSM allows correct/incorrect naming of

syndromes and leaves us with the *illusion* of quantification, then it traps us into thinking we are doing something we are not. This is especially true of the illusory "quantification" notion.

Quantifying can be accurate, objective, mathematical measurements or can be described in terms like "more" or "less," which is quite different. These words sound equally objective, but they are not. So we are not measuring, we are using "measurement-speak." Any "quantifications" are not so and only make sense in common psychiatric parlance among psychiatrists or others, for example.

Still, whatever we may criticize in the field of psychiatry, it has also provided psychology, social work, and counseling fields with a diagnostic system they lacked.

Psychology, Social Work, and Counseling

Social Work and Counseling have no alternative to the DSM, though there are DSM-derived surveys or other systems to measure mental health functioning, as does the field of psychology. It may not be well known, but the field of psychology has produced an enormous number of tests, measurements, and theories. Its production is so enormous that others pale into lesser significance.

Other fields' practitioners cannot typically employ psychological measuring devices, since many are only available for administration by psychologists. One might consider why psychologists have created so much valuable data. The answer: *It is in the nature of their education.*

Part of the dynamic is that psychologists essentially study psychological issues, and others study *their* field's issues. More importantly, social workers on an MSW level don't require a thesis;

neither do master's level counselors, psychiatrists, or other MDs, as part of their normal medical education.

Psychologists on the doctoral level and, in some schools on a master's level, are required to produce a thesis, and those theses advance the field's developments; thus the geometric rate of advance. When I was in graduate school in the early 1960s the field of psychology doubled its production every eight years!

Chapter Five

DSM TRADITIONAL CLASSIFICATION
AND NEW VARIANTS

THE TRADITIONAL DSM HAS BEEN PUBLISHED in many versions that were modified with the latest thinking on diagnosis and classifications. There are different views within the psychiatric community regarding each version's value. This discussion was engaged earlier in this text.

The present discussion involves two differing approaches that are essentially moving in a similar direction from different points. One is neurophysiological and brain-based, the other psychologically and statistically based, incorporating factor analysis.

Frances's suggestion of developing research to provide the biological basis of normal and pathological behaviors has begun. Dr. Cozolino's work in neurobiology is the type of inquiry he is proposing, and this line of research is exceedingly admirable and state-of-the-art.

The alternate format for investigation and clarification of the DSM is factor analysis, a statistic that provides assessment of many aspects of, in this case, human pathological behavior. Prior statistical assessments were more one-dimensional than multi-dimensional.

"The current diagnostic system for personality disorders (PD) has a number of problems that may require a thorough revision for DSM-V. This article (a) outlines problems with the current taxonomy that suggest the need for a different approach to PD diagnosis, that preserves the strengths of the current system while addressing some inherent weaknesses; (b) discusses key issues that must be addressed in moving toward DSM-V, such as revising the distinction between Axis I and Axis II and combining categorical and dimensional diagnosis; and (c) describes a prototype matching approach to diagnosis, which we believe has the potential to be both psychometrically sound and faithful to the clinical data.

"Theory and research have suggested that the personality disorders contained within the American Psychiatric Association's *Diagnostic and Statistical Manual of Mental Disorders* (*DSM-IV-TR*) can be understood as maladaptive variants of the personality traits included within the five-factor model (FFM). The current meta-analysis of FFM personality disorder research both replicated and extended the 2004 work of Saulsman and Page. The five-factor model and personality disorder, through a facet level analysis, provides a more specific and nuanced description of each *DSM-IV-TR* personality disorder. The empirical FFM profiles generated for each personality disorder were generally congruent at the facet level with hypothesized FFM translations of the *DSM-IV-TR* personality disorders. However, notable exceptions to the hypotheses did occur and even some findings that were consistent with FFM theory could be said to be instrument specific" (Saulsman & Page, 2004, pp. 1055-1085).

Factor Analysis As An Alternative Approach

The DSMs have ben very helpful in verbally categorizing pathological behaviors and syndromes in individuals for many years.

Though words can be carefully chosen to reflect syndromes accurately, words are not enough to move psychiatry on to higher levels of precision and prediction from nominal to ordinal, to interval, and, if possible, ratio.

The DSMs, even now with the DSM-V version, describe personality disorders as, "an enduring pattern of inner experience and behavior that deviates markedly from the expectations of the individuals['] culture is pervasive and inflexible. . .and leads to distress and impairment" (DSM-IV-TR 1994, p. 629).

Blais (1997, pp. 388-394) notes, "Either way, as the DSM criteria for personality disorders have been developed from clinical experience rather than empirical investigation, it is time these concepts of trait atypicality, cross–situational consistency, and negative consequence, plus trait combination and trait-environment fit, be assessed empirically to uncover what distinguishes pathological personality from [just] extreme personality."

A second major issue is the distinction between categorical and dimensional systems of organizing and perceiving how personality disorders exist, specifically how far one goes in judging where the extremity of that personality disorder ends.

Consider narcissistic personality disorder. How far does one need to go with "self-love" before it leaves the normal realm and enters the pathological?

Essentially, the *categorical* aspect says the end is a specific point, and the *dimensional* says there is a shading of description without defined borders. You can probably see that words are inadequate to the task—the essence of the DSM quandary. This is a great example of why and how each of any system's accuracy is challenged—*if you're employing words, you are limited to very subjective interpretations.*

The way out in one regard is statistical; the second is biological. We'll deal with the statistical first. It is important to note that this tradition is not part of psychiatry, social work, or counseling, as it clearly is in psychology.

From its beginning, with Wundt and experimental psychology, numbers preceded and dominated words. Psychology was on a different and more fruitful track.

The Five Factor Model of Personality is more accurate and predictable than the DSMs in describing personality disorders. The purpose of the Five Factor research is to improve the DSM assessment process.

Factor analysis was introduced briefly in the introduction to this book. Five Factor Model researchers began with the ten personality disorders as described in any DSM: Paranoid, Schizoid, Schizotypal, Antisocial, Borderline, Histrionic, Narcissistic, Avoidant, Dependent, and Obsessive-Compulsive.

Each of these was paired with the five personality dimensions of the Five Factor Model: Neuroticism, Extraversion, Openness to Experience, Agreeableness, and Conscientiousness. It is important to note these FF terms are not the same as DSM terms, because they were derived from statistical analysis.

The analysis evaluates behaviors that are *independent* of someone's assumptions—any person or mental health professional's—of what may be connected to verbal personality descriptions.

We should be clear, again, that we have a great debt to the field of psychiatry for its first attempt to organize and employ a descriptive system that is independent of later improvements we are introducing.

Locating behaviors that are *independent* means *independent from subjective labels*, and that thereby offer a baseline from which to judge the accuracy of those labels and move closer to a more accurate and thorough system.

In brief, this factor analytic evaluation does not mean the FF Model dimensions necessarily reject prior DSM labels; it only indicates which of them "loads" more or less on those labels so we can be more comfortable in using the newer terms for diagnosis and treatment.

I will not be presenting the personality dimension tables, since they are long involved lists of numbers in percentages for each of the FF dimensions. The greater the percentage, the greater the purity of each dimension, and the more useful and accurate that dimension is to the DSM labels.

Quoting from Saulsman and Page (2005, pp. 1055-1085), "Schizoid and Schizotypal personality disorders are characterized by negative relationships with Extraversion, with Schizotypal personality disorder showing further positive associations with Neuroticism and negative associations with Agreeableness.

"Paranoid and Borderline personality disorders are characterized by both positive correlations with Neuroticism and negative correlations with Agreeableness, with Paranoid being more related to Agreeableness and Borderline being more related to Neuroticism." Of course these quotes are offered only to provide a hint of how the factor analytic system of evaluation works in refining DSM labels.

A Biological Approach—Cozolino

I have quoted Louis Cozolino's (2002) work as an early example of this system earlier in this volume.

Cozolino introduces his ideas by noting, "Because it was so scientifically and politically difficult to study the brain, Freud chose to study the mind. . . . [He] postulated that what we witness of consciousness and unconsciousness processing is reflected in the neural architecture of the brain and central nervous system" (Schore, 1997, pp. 841-867). "Freud became obsessed with the idea of constructing a model of the mind in terms of its neurobiological mechanisms."

Cozolino's position is that the brain develops from reptilian to paleomammalian on its way to becoming human. "The result is that a great deal of learning takes place before we have the necessary cortical systems for conscious awareness and memory" (2002, p. 12). (As an aside, note that "conscious awareness" is the only kind there is; "unconscious awareness" is an oxymoron, like "jumbo shrimp." So even first-rate investigators can misuse words.)

Neuronal development is slow, and in our early years we are functioning with mostly inherited genetic "hardware," though as he notes, "70% of our genetic structure is added after birth" (p.

22). He views psychotherapy as a means of enhancing neural networks, creating plasticity and neurogenesis—a growth and change process.

He quotes Orlinsky and Howard, who found "factors that related to psychotherapeutic success were the quality of the emotional connection between the patient and [the] therapist [and are] far more important than the theoretical orientation of the therapist" (p. 40). Extremely interesting and insightful—that what we believe matters very much, matters very little.

This approach elucidates the brain's neural networks and provides a very different means of explaining the brain's functions. More importantly for our purposes, it allows a far better means of diagnosis and treatment than any of the DSM versions. Factor analysis parallels this process from a non-biological perspective.

Together, then, we have the merging of two long-standing traditions—medical and psychological. While statistical, since factor analysis is mathematical, it is also a significant component of psychology, unlike the other mental health fields we've discussed.

This is another example of the continuing development in two ancient fields, each of which had to await changes in other fields for them to progress.

Nothing is as new as we often think. It is our job to know our pasts and to continue them with some small deviations that interpret issues when they seem to stop, as explained in the book *The Structure of Scientific Revolutions* (Kuhn, 1962), which I will discuss later.

Chapter Six

TRANSITION FROM PSYCHOLOGY
TO CHEMICAL DEPENDENCE

A T THIS POINT, WE CAN FINALLY enter the alcohol/drug (A/D) fields and their formal beginning in the twentieth-century with Bill W., Dr. Bob, and the Alcoholics Anonymous approach.

My attempt in this treatise is to demonstrate how long, ancient, and sophisticated the academic and applied fields of philosophy and psychology were—and all well before the formal field of chemical dependence began.

Although there was no rapprochement or merging of the two fields earlier, it did occur when psychological and psychiatric professionals began to evaluate how *their* fields could assess and change C/D treatment.

Alcoholics Anonymous

AA was begun by alcoholics and for alcoholics, by those who agreed that there was moral and spiritual deformation of the alcoholic, and that the 12 Steps–12 Traditions proposed would put them on the road to recovery.

Begun in 1935 by Bill Wilson and Dr. Bob, and others who were alcoholics themselves, it was designed to be free and self- supporting, with no connections to any other organization. Its simple goal was to help alcoholics achieve and maintain sobriety. It should be recalled that Carl Jung, the psychoanalyst, aided the start of this approach.

Recent denials by the main organization of the "religious" aspects of AA are true to the extent it has no formal relationship with any organized religion, especially non-Christian ones. However, the messianic style of many members would have one believe otherwise. Belief in a "higher power" is identical to a God, and the member is encouraged to seek one's higher power in anything or anyone. The number of Steps—Traditions—is twelve, similar to the twelve apostles of Christ.

The therapeutic value of this approach seems to be part of the overall technique of taking excess pressure off the alcoholic and placing it outside the self, where it is more manageable. This, in turn, adds to the change from self-interest and isolation to interaction with others, a dynamic that is anathema to a CD person.

As a member progresses, they accept a "sponsor" and call that person, at a frequency of from daily to whenever, to ask for help and check in. The sponsor assists the "sponsee" with readings, advice, and encouragement to read "The Big Book," (AA), attend meetings, and pursue the "Twelve Steps."

The Steps are essentially a survey of aspects of a CD person's life issues; Step Four is the process of completing this list with the sponsor's help, which tends to make the member more aware of issues from their life that affect them in dealing with others. AA has other chapters, such as Al-Anon. Their development over time shows an organization responding to the many areas of difficulty in a CD person's life, including marital and child issues. There are periodic "retreats," again remarkably similar to Christianity's religious retreats.

The main issue is AA has become more and more therapeutic over time, with positive and negative outcomes for its members. It should be noted AA's main organization and its principles are not responsible for *some* of its followers' practices.

The positive features include greater tolerance for the CD person, especially because AA has implied, since near its inception, that there is a familial component in alcoholism treatment. The number of sponsors who are more therapeutically sophisticated has increased as members partake of traditional and CD psychotherapy, as well as medicines, themselves.

This has led those particular members and sponsors to sometimes offer advice to sponsees that is beyond their capacity to legitimately offer. This help is carried to the point of diagnosing people and recommending whether they should or should not take medications, and continue or terminate psychotherapy.

This practice is a function of the membership of some AA meetings. There is need for careful investigation of AA meetings by the prospective member with regard to their "medical" stance and advice giving, just as when one chooses a meeting according to age and the characteristics of members there, i.e., whether they are mostly working, mostly established with their sobriety, etc.

Clinical Psychological/Psychiatric Treatment: The Beginning Of Dual Diagnosis—Mental Health

The assumption, derived from psychoanalysis, was that CD individuals had hidden motivations that drove their addiction and that, if these were resolved, the individual could be free of their addiction.

The CD individual's continued use of chemicals, motivation, and being under the influence at treatment sessions were often regarded as a problem that interfered with the search for insight and therefore required the therapist to terminate or not even begin treatment, because the patient was "resistant."

Alternatively, the patient was seen as addicted, and treatment would proceed in spite of their use until control could be established by the patient.

The fallacy was in:

1. Assuming addiction was only, or primarily, driven by a personal motivation to drink, or,

2. That the individual had chosen to drink for reasons of character deformation. The notion that addiction was driven by genes and their stepchild brain hormones was to await advancement in these fields.

Government Funding—The '60s

Although the federal government provided scattered funding for counseling to states and cities in the 1960s, it was initially sporadic and not very effective, for several reasons.

Besides the administrative costs being deducted from such grants by local governments, there was the unavoidable fact that no one was sure what would *be* effective, and for which drug users/addicts. Additionally, for the first time in many years, middle-class adolescents were affected, and this too altered the pattern of funding—it was increased. To its credit, the federal government invested in many approaches.

Among those:

- Local counseling agencies run by mental health personnel
- AA-type offshoots
- A chemical approach with Antabuse (Disulfram) for alcohol
- Methadone for opiates
- Inpatient therapeutic communities like Synanon and Daytop

Opiates were the most dangerous, since addicts were dying, especially from injectable heroin. Cannabis and hallucinogens, which were on the rise, were more complicated to treat, so monies for research appeared. In the interim, such individuals were accepted to therapeutic communities (if the therapeutic community's census permitted) and intensive outpatient CD, or mental health practitioners.

Chapter Seven

THERAPEUTIC COMMUNITIES

HERAPEUTIC COMMUNITIES (TCs) EXISTED prior to their appearance in the field of CD treatment. The earliest communities are attributed to the Alexandrian Egyptians, where sick members of the community could be helped—curing their soul—by living with others.

In the U.S. and Europe, they were fostered as places for treatment, particularly psychiatric, in foreign countries. One could broaden the definition to include those that "hippies" inhabited; the latter were essentially social enclaves, not treatment facilities, places to share expenses and personal relationships.

The therapeutic communities in foreign countries treated those with long-term psychiatric diagnoses; there also were communities for training regimens for professionals, such as those run by the Tavistock Clinic. These employed social psychoanalytic theories, e.g., Wilfred Bion (1959), Melanie Klein, and Boris Astrachan's, to provide insight into people's relationships with regard to employment of control and power.

This specific approach was applied to a therapeutic community called Liberty Village, at which I was the clinical psychologist/ clinical director, which I will discuss later.

Synanon was established in San Francisco, California, in the late 1950s by Chuck Dederich (De Leon, 2000). He was a recovering alcoholic and, along with others, developed a TC for the purpose of treating drug-addicted individuals. Dederich employed a set of principles similar to those that governed AA, but with changes necessary to accommodate the TC group-treatment philosophy.

Whereas AA established higher power, self-examination and mutual self-help principles, Synanon replaced these with a secular ideology and reliance upon self-determination and individual responsibility.

In several respects, this change reflects a more cognitive shift, not unlike that occurring in the field of academic and clinical psychology. This phenomenon of many different investigators tapping the same well of ideas was labeled the *Zeitgeist* ("spirit" in German), noted by the famous experimental psychologist E.G. Boring (1929).

The greatest difference between AA and Synanon, or other TCs to my mind, was the TC society's role of:

- Public viewing of an individual's behavior and its consequences, sometimes with devastating implications for the individual
- Modeling of desirable and undesirable behaviors for adoption by the CD individual

Daytop Village and Phoenix House (Phoenix, the Greek mythical bird that rose to life from its ashes) were begun in New York City after Synanon was established but had very similar treatment principles and philosophies.

Liberty Village—A T.C. Paradigm

The following exposition of a TC is my recollection of the workings of a therapeutic community with my involvement from 1971 to 1973. I am, however, aware the specifics I am referring to may be a function of the time, and particularly the state, of the CD field during that period. My goal is to show changes in treatment approaches and theories over time, and I will compare other TC models as well with those in operation today.

Liberty Village was established by a group of recovering people from Daytop Village, before my time there, who were employed by the Board of the New Jersey Regional Drug Abuse Agency to provide this "new" treatment approach. The facility had its main site in Jersey City, New Jersey, on property that faced the Statue of Liberty and where Liberty State Park is located today.

Additional properties existed in the main part of Jersey City proper—Christopher House, and Cedar Grove-Liberty House I—the Narcotic Addict Rehabilitation Act (NARA) program to deal with those released from prison and ready to reenter society.

Liberty Village had a maximum total population of about two hundred inpatients, and those in treatment would be there for about eighteen months, though this varied with program stages and individual development. Initially, residents could have no contact with their families or significant others and, later, received gradually extended time away from the facility as they improved.

Since this program served residents of Hudson and Essex Counties, there also were about ten Outreach Centers that provided outpatient treatment and acted as intake centers for referral to inpatient treatment. The outpatient population there varied from hundreds to about a thousand, depending on the flow of new patients.

Liberty Village initially had the following facilities on the main grounds or "property":
- The main residence for about two hundred inpatients
  - A twenty-four-hour medical detox and treatment facility with a medical doctor, psychiatrist, psychologist, and nurses
  - A "school" with teachers to assist residents with educational and career issues
  - A social work staff to deal with residents' non-residential issues and relationships

LV's Stages of Treatment
- Detox—medical detox—for a few days up to two weeks
- Main Residence, or "House," for about nine months to one year
- Re-Entry (to society) on a half-time basis. At LV, there was no separate halfway house, so residents lived in the dorms.

The development of this community is instructive, and I served as clinical psychologist, later Clinical Director, and was privileged to observe and fully participate in this process.

A patient came to LV via the outreach centers of LV and other places throughout the state and other states. They were charged a fee for treatment if they came from outside the two counties. NARA patient treatment was funded by the federal government. All "residents," as they were called, were evaluated medically and psychologically and, when cleared, entered the treatment residence.

The residential staff reminded the resident that they were at the bottom of the totem pole, and that its philosophy was to replace the resident's defective lifestyle/personality with a healthier one. It is relevant to note that the population was typically 60–80 percent male and about 20 percent, maximum, female. The implications of this imbalance will be addressed later.

T.C. Treatment Approaches

Synanon's use of Alexandrian Egypt's therapeutic community approach was present at LV as well as at other facilities, but the differences among TCs were often quite varied. LV had a basic TC approach, modeled directly after Daytop Village of course, that included the following:

- Almost exclusively group treatment
- Peer support and "adoption" (a resident with more time in treatment "adopted" the new resident)
- Learning experiences:
  Loss of privileges
  Signs and "haircuts" (verbal reprimands/shaved heads)
- Structured daily schedule
- Non-residential activities

To focus on each, in order, the group treatment approach had the advantages of allowing many to be treated by a few, and of allowing residents to see others resolving or not resolving their issues, and what the consequences of each were.

To have a few provide treatment was economical, along with the "one size fits all" approach that permitted easy assimilation of information. I am aware that there were adjustments to the "one-size" model by individual staff, but these were rare and not terribly different from the mainstream.

This one-size approach is similar to AA's adages, such as "keep it green" (i.e., keep it new—remember where you came from). CD people loved, and still love, these facile, even glib statements. The number of nicknames for drugs, for example, is legion, with thousands of them for perhaps a hundred drugs.

It reflects the narcissism and grandiosity of the typical CD person to have a sickness, or a situation, that is beyond mortal men's and women's ability to resolve. One LV residential director was married on the property on Valentine's Day—a hint of "royalty."

When a group member is told how to resolve an issue, it is advice the group leader has learned to provide, perhaps to the complete exclusion of other advice and approaches. The resident also adopted this approach because they know nothing—KISS—AA's "Keep it simple, stupid." To simplify can be good, as a first step especially, but the problem is that treatment may, and often does, *stay* simple.

Besides simplicity, the group approach was employed by others who have had only *their* own experience, taught by mentors who have had only *their* experience, leading to premature closure.

The group approach is also "cognitive," as noted earlier in this chapter with Dederich's TC principles, but a cognitive approach is easier to perform and very relevant to the early stage of a resident who, upon entry into residence, is still enduring secondary and tertiary detoxing and cognitively confused.

One of the shortcomings of this overly cognitive approach is premature closure, e.g., chiding a resident about abuse of females in and out of residence with "Disrespect is a no-no." The need for control is evident in a TC when feedback must be stated in this way; however, it only enforces external controls and only temporarily suppresses the desire to act out.

This is treatment from the "outside in" rather than the "inside out"—a phenomenon we will see repeated in all later treatment discussions in the field of addiction as well as psychology in general, represented by the insight/analytic vs. cognitive/behavioral approaches.

Reflective approaches would arouse more feeling and lead to a risk of acting out but could also lead to internal, rather than external, controls (see Locus of Control and Internalizing and Externalizing studies, discussed later).

This reflective approach could not be employed by the recovery staff because they knew nothing of it; it was also alien to their format. It could not have been employed in the early phase of treatment because of the risk of acting out; its appropriate use would have been later in the program.

The central issue seems to be, although treatment of an external type was necessary for control of the community, *its continued use to the exclusion of other approaches* severely limited a resident's development, which in turn unnecessarily threatened the community's stability. The residential staff's view is, if the residents improve, then there is nothing to fix.

Clarity in such discussions always requires determination of

what the goals of any treatment approach are. Some are obvious:
- · Control of the resident(s) for the sake of a stable community
- · Need to set examples for acting-out people, so they would not emulate negative behaviors
- · Enforcing the cardinal rules—sex, drugs, rebellion, disrespect
- · Prevention of influx of drugs, and reduction of A.M.A. (Against Medical Advice) discharges.

A prime illustrative example of the effects of treatment and their consequences is probably best presented via the residential life cycle of a fledgling staff member who moves through the residential treatment program. It will involve us with the goals above.

The "Expediter"

The term "expediter" describes a resident who has improved sufficiently over time to assume some staff responsibilities. He (almost always a male) could be called a "gofer" in other settings. His job is to do the bidding of more senior (and paid) staff, to oversee residents and report their behaviors, perhaps to run groups, transport residents to various visits outside the facility, etc.

The resident-to-expediter process is instructive, but it should be noted that not all residents could become expediters, because then there would be no residents! An expediter's job is partly to oversee residents' behavior and to report it to staff. The resident's treatment path is externally controlled, and the greater his assimilation of staff–congruent behaviors, the greater the likelihood of advancement through the program and toward the role of expediter.

This degree of staff-congruence in a "street" person was not always straightforward, of course. Residents were, and are, a combination of many personality types—inadequate, anti-social, socio-pathic, narcissistic, impulsive, and rarely, psychotic, etc., with and without mood disorders and A.D.D. Honesty was not their strong suit! In fact, the resident would often manipulate staff by appearing to be congruent in order to advance. In this respect the process mirrored what had been done to survive outside the facility.

There was also compliance by staff with negative contracting—"I'll do this for you, if you do that for me." Negative contracting occurred between the expediter and the resident as well. To the extent this occurred, it vitiated the effect of positive change and reinforced the residents' and expediter's view that honesty and consistency are illusions.

An example of this is an expediter negatively contracting with a woman in residence who was agreeable to having sex with him, which was negatively beneficial for both. He was sexually satisfied and exercised his special status, and she continued her control of men via sexual favors that led to self-debasement.

On the other hand, if an expediter were *honestly* congruent, he could also become the inheritor of a less demanding course through the residence. This process often protected the expediter from experiencing what needed to be done for him and could, and did, lead to problems for him and the residence. Although it may not have been intended, the expediter could leave the standard resident's path early and "graduate" to re-entry.

Women

The differential numbers of men and women in residence was noted earlier. Women comprised about 20 percent of the population and were, by definition, outnumbered. Women were less likely to be arrested because they committed less violent crimes and behaviors, and were therefore less likely to *need* residential treatment. They assumed a less dominant role on the street and could also have been the girlfriend or prostitute of men, some of whom were in residence with them.

Women were less interested in seeking help, and when they did enter a residence, they were more likely to "split" (leave A.M.A.) the facility. They were not always fragile and in need of protection, however. They were co-dependent upon male residents they either knew from the street, or chose to relate in this way to men they didn't know. In either case, they were sabotaging their treatment from its onset.

The desire to depend upon a man for strength and sustenance was often balanced by the desire to control her destiny without him. When environmental changes/stressors occurred, she would choose the better alternative at the time. It seems female dynamics were not as simple as the program's structure assumed.

Given the set of dynamics between men and women, it was a major challenge for residential staff to modify. The dilemma was, the staff may not have resolved their own issues regarding sexuality or other male/female behaviors. As always, the treatment staff's mental health affected what they did, for and against residents and others.

As noted, women rarely ran groups, except for Female Group, where residents could discuss their issues. In all other groups, women were merely members and often used and abused by men. In some instances, women split when forced to deal with issues they thought had no good exit strategy.

They tended to have a higher A.M.A. rate and were more likely to see mutual difficulties as primarily their fault, not their male counterparts'. The obverse was that women who split would often encourage men to split with them.

When an expediter broke a cardinal rule, he was demoted to a resident status. This was intended to create anxiety and anger toward him as a consequence. The diminution of self-esteem was an intended aspect of treatment for all residents. However, there was less support for its reciprocal, the *enhancement* of self-esteem.

It was always interesting and confounding that people with terrible self-esteem would need to be built up by being torn down. Related to this is the mental stability and mettle of staff. When a cardinal rule was broken and consequences were chosen, the staff's demeanor was often tense and suggested an insult had been promulgated by the resident toward *them*.

In those instances where more restraint and good judgment were displayed, the staff person was typically more intact and less threatened. The Tavistock system of power sharing in groups is relevant here and will be discussed later in this chapter.

Breaking rules required consequences and revealed an aspect of good "parenting" by residential staff. However, the nature of punishment ran the gamut from reasonable to absurd.

For example, if someone had behaved like a baby by acting out, such as crying, having a tantrum, etc., they would be provided with a learning experience. A likely one was to wear a "sign"—similar to those worn by out-of-work people advertising a business or asking for a job on the street during the Great Depression. It would proclaim, *I am a baby—treat me that way,* and they would be dressed in a baby's frilly outfit, with a baby bottle in their hand.

Residents would enjoy playing this game of debasement as part of the consequence for their behavior, which expressed their own anxiety about not being chosen for such an act, as well as to demonstrate their incorporation of the house's (staff's) cultural prerogatives.

This is consistent with the rationale of the TC, in that there is the intended replacement of the dysfunctional self with a more functional one. From an "outside-in" perspective, it seems sensible. However, as effective as it is with brute-force control of behavior in the short run, it leaves untouched the long-term behavior change one needs to achieve.

Further, and this is important, all approaches have the central goal of drug abstinence, but *enhanced approaches address the changes necessary to live a life as well.* The parallel to the "dry drunk" term from AA's lexicon is legitimate—someone who doesn't drink but lives a secluded, brittle existence.

I am reminded of one person who attends one or more daily AA meetings with many years of sobriety but lives in the basement of his three-story home next to the furnace, with the floors above him as empty as his life.

As might be imagined, residents would respond differentially to this experience according to their personality type. Inadequate types would probably withdraw in hurt and may even split, because of the embarrassment of exposure. An antisocial type would be more likely to get even later, or outright refuse compliance, leading to a more severe consequence.

Other learning experiences included "haircuts." These involved shaving the heads of male residents to diminish them, as well as have the intent of taking the resident's pride—his hair. This procedure echoes its biblical roots with Samson and Delilah.

Those who tried to split and were caught, on at least one occasion that I witnessed, had been provided with time in a walk-in refrigerator (for food storage) to remind the resident how "cold" the outside world was and that they'd be better off staying in the TC.

These experiences were legitimized in the eyes of staff because they would stop a resident from leaving and perhaps killing themselves; the intent was laudable and appropriate, the means highly questionable.

As mentioned in an earlier chapter, another resident had nocturnal enuresis. This was not tolerable in the dorms, so he was one of the residents slated to wear a baby sign and dress. I was staff psychologist at the time, and the residential staff asked for my help. The opportunity was welcomed as a potential rapprochement between recovering and "straight" (non-CD) staff.

I might add that I had known one or two LV staff before being hired, and this made it easier for me to be welcomed as a friend and someone who knew the street personality well.

The resident was seen medically and psychiatrically before deciding to employ this approach. I purchased a behavioral device from Sears to modify his enuresis.

The device employed Mowrer's learning theory. It had two sheets of metal, connected at the ends that, when placed on a bed, were then attached to a battery and a bell. A bed sheet was placed between them and would not allow the bell to ring unless the bed sheet was wet, thereby completing the electrical circuit. When the resident became enuretic during the night, the bell went off, and he would then use the bathroom, wash his body and replace the bed sheet.

In about ten days his enuresis terminated. The staff was impressed, as was I. Now they were aware of other approaches that worked, much better than the negative consequences of a sign or haircut. Some staff were supportive of this new approach, but others, as we might expect, believed it was changing a tried-and-true approach, again, a parallel to AA intransigence.

The conservative nature of a more close-minded person not open to demonstrated change strove to maintain a tradition that sometimes got in its own way. These staff differences—essentially people differences—were to play a significant role in the future of LV's treatment modifications, which lay ahead.

Peer Support and "Adoption"

In the normal course of events, a new resident was assigned to an "older" (in treatment time) resident and perhaps one who had similar difficulties. The peer provided directions, advice, and generally played a role similar to that of the expediter for the house. This idea is effective because the new resident leans on the older one and has a better chance of staying and changing—a wise policy.

Structured Daily Activities

The residence was run in "boot camp" fashion with:
- Early rising and hygienic activities
- Breakfast and cleanup, including kitchen duties, if that was one's job
- Morning meeting—whole house
- Groups

- Visits to medical, psychological, and educational personnel, sometimes in lieu of a particular group on that day and time
- Lunch with clean up
- Groups
- Visits or classes with non-residential staff
- Supper with cleanup
- Groups
- Downtime with TV or relaxation
- Bedtime

Weekends usually involved passes with time away from the facility with family, friends, and peers. For those who agreed with the AA idea of avoiding "people, places, and things" but were not ready, a peer would accompany them on the pass. Those without passes enjoyed visits from family, or significant others, if they qualified.

Given the spectrum of activities in and out of residence, and on and off the property, a resident's life was routine but active. This high level of activity is a salient aspect of the TC and one that accommodates the busy and negative-seeking minds of the typical resident. Additionally, the number of behaviors that could be observed by residential and professionally trained staff was vast, and allowed them to validate hypotheses about a resident's diagnosis, issues, and recommendations.

Residential Staff/Professional Culture

Each TC, at least in the early days of the field, had built-in suspicions between these two groups. The residential staff members were all recovering from CD, and some of the professional staff often not only did not use drugs but never had.

As such, the recovering staff felt ambivalent—not having achieved as much as the professional staff in their education and status, such as it was. Conversely, residential staff were feeling empathetic, because they knew exactly what the residents were going through, and what they needed via this treatment model. They were the practitioners of the main treatment modality—professionals were ancillary staff.

Although the professional staff generally agreed with this proposition, there were also differences between those non-CD staff who were traditionally trained in mental health and those who came from formal religious training, the Catholic priesthood in this case.

There were legitimate differences—traditional staff had never been exposed to a TC with its bold and aggressive style that just looked wrong. They had been taught to be supportive and empathetic, while recovering staff knew better.

CD people could manipulate an empathetic style, and they did. On the other hand, the "control" approach, working from the "outside-in," didn't allow the freedom to employ much empathy. It could be argued that the need for control was a responsible but, as noted earlier, also a limiting factor.

This treatment style arose from the confines of the culture. It was a hands-on work in progress that grew out of a core of battle-tested ideas. In retrospect, every system can be critiqued—and this one was—by many people, including me.

A Revised Treatment Modality

After about a year, I saw many difficulties with the treatment style and outcomes that could be changed—as well as the need to maintain the TC structure and its valid aspects. The dilemma was how to implement an approach that, to our knowledge, had never been discussed, least of all put into practice; the year was 1972.

Additionally, the house directors would not have tolerated changes they believed fixed something that wasn't broken. Residential staffs in many TCs I visited and/or knew well—in New York, New Jersey, Pennsylvania, and Florida, and probably across the country—typically responded by pointing to the success of their approach, as people in AA did, and still do.

However, there were no good long-term statistics, and their defense echoed what is still touted today—that, when a person fails, they're "not ready" or haven't "hit bottom." This certainly is true in many cases, but not generally. The reciprocal view was that we needed to find a modality broad enough to include such people.

In this respect, the TC *chose* whom it could deal with and change. Again, one could argue that all modalities employ such choosing, and that it is wise to do so. However, in a TC—literally a community, a small city—the givens of the historical accidents of race, gender, and culture controlled the treatment options.

The Problems

- A largely white male staff
- A largely male residential population
- A demeaning culture
- The assumption that one could dismantle a personality and replace it with a "better" one
- The separation of recovering and professional staff
- The recovering staff's pervasive criticism of straight staff to

residents, encouraging a culture of distrust and disrespect that maintained the addict's lifestyle, opinions, and potential for relapse

· Most importantly, the lack of an enhanced program that broadened both treatment and vocational opportunities

I had crystallized ideas over the first year and discussed them with select, i.e., open-minded, recovering, and straight staff. Although I firmly believed they would work, the central figure to convince was the Director of LV, Jerry Feulner. He had been a priest before leaving the priesthood in the 1960s and was very willing to consider ideas different from his own. It was a bit easier because he had promoted me from clinical psychologist to clinical director and trusted what I thought.

The Proposed Solution

Replace the white residential director with a black man, but one who had the requisite temperament and knowledge. The black man chosen would not be accepted easily by residential staff, even those who were black, even in the racially conflicted '60s, because he was not one of them, i.e., not in the TC tradition—the very reason he was chosen.

Admit more women. This could be achieved but would need to be preceded by a change in attitude and treatment format. The central goal was not primarily to increase the female census, but to create a more effective treatment modality for them.

Drop the demeaning aspects of treatment—signs, haircuts, and other inappropriate behaviors—but establish appropriate learning experiences and consequences.

Implement a holistic treatment modality, which could hit the ground running and develop immediate success that inspired confidence. In the TC world, resistance to change is strong, and a new idea has a very small window for acceptance.

The therapy approach would be a reflective one that allowed a broader view, and discussion of, problems. It would have the benefit of the "pairs" therapists noted below.

It would be humanistic to allow greater involvement of residents to express honest and even negative information to be dealt with in a more effective manner. It would retain learning experiences, but ones more closely *related to the particular conflict expressed* within the resident's behavior.

It removed expediters from being quasi-residential treatment staff. In fact, no resident would have this level of responsibility during their treatment experience. Each resident would instead learn how to be helpful to others by observing, participating, and learning *within the group.*

Any resident could assume the role of helper to others—the hallmark of TCs—but would not have a therapeutic role memorialized in the structure. The difficulty with this role assumption within the old TC was that *it introduced a power- struggle sharing that the unstable resident was not ready to assume.*

Power sharing was at the core of TC treatment; it was the fulcrum that moved everything. To use it without fully understanding it, without having recognized it and resolved it within oneself, led to a plethora of difficulties for everyone. *One of its most detrimental aspects was the programming its non-resolution created for relapse.*

Lastly, LV recovering staff viewed their job as *Re-Habilitation*, but this implies returning someone to a prior state of more effective functioning. In fact, some street addicts were so primitive they *never* had been capable of adequate socialization. In this respect, the job was more accurately described as Habilitation.

Blend the boundaries between residential and straight staffs. Specifically, I suggested offering recovering staff members the opportunity to join the new modality. I would hire new staff that would be *paired* as "therapists" for groups. Each pair was composed of one man and one woman, one recovering person and one professionally trained (minimum bachelor's degree, but master's preferred).

Continue clinical rounds at each facility—main property at LV, Christopher House, National Addict Rehabilitation Act (N.A.R.A.)—and have treatment pairs attend to discuss difficult issues, as opposed to having more senior staff leaders make decisions for them.

The end result of this pairing would be not only to end the staff separation but, mainly, to model integrated relationships for residents to emulate and trust— in and out of the house. The emulation would be male/female, straight/recovering, educated/less educated, street/privileged, as well as the differences in personalities.

Implement Enhancements directed toward life outside the residence. The most glaring shortcoming of any TC was the vocational component. The plan was to dovetail a vocational evaluation and a hands-on work experience *on the property*, with the approval and help of the New Jersey Division of Vocational Rehabilitation. The person who ran the program had a master's degree in vocational rehabilitation.

Another aspect of vocational training is the lack of knowledge about it possessed by the average resident. Avoiding the same old job or career is similar to AA's "people, places, and things," but without marketable skills, one's job was a detriment for sobriety.

Vocational information would allow staff to know the limits of work capacity and quality a resident possessed. This would have bearing on their behavior in and out of the residence, as well as improving a resident's self-esteem. Residents who were not effective in the residence might be "stars" in vocational training.

How To Introduce Change Without Detriment

In all of our opinions, leadership staff in the residence would not accept the change in treatment and would possibly negatively influence the minds of residents who could be hurt by leaving prematurely. Our primary concern was for the residents, not for this opportunity for change.

Jerry Feulner and other professional staff, including key board members, agreed with my ideas and wanted them implemented. In an earlier chapter, I noted the TC concept in Britain, for treatment as well as training. Prior to assuming the position at LV, I was on the full-time faculty at New York Medical College, in the doctoral psychology program at the New School Graduate Faculty, and in psychoanalysis at Columbia.

As a corollary to psychoanalysis, I participated in Tavistock (Tavy) experiences, which examined power in social groups in several life situations. Feulner agreed that he and the rest of the administrative staff would benefit from participating in a weekend Tavy. This solidified everyone and improved our relationships for the residential changes to come.

The Tavy staff, who were from Columbia and Yale (the Institute for the Applied Study of Social Systems). IASOSS also consulted to our staff on-site and provided us with resolution of issues which would have limited our conversion of the residence as well.

A corporate-style replacement of residence leadership was also considered—giving written notice to employees who were being let go, and a month or so to find a replacement while they continued to administer, would be far too damaging for the residents. By design, a "coup" was chosen.

On a Monday, the residential leaders were called to Jerry Feulner's office and told of the plan, provided with severance, and told they would be accompanied to their offices, where they would remove their belongings and leave the property. It was later found that our fears of negative influence by them were justified.

Implementation

Without further elaboration, the new treatment format was put into effect and worked as well or better than most expected. The tone of the residence changed dramatically in ways we had anticipated—initial freedom and relaxation of the rules, followed by the need to tighten control, and we did.

Residents preferred the change, and group therapeutic exchanges were more real and effective. Time periods in treatment were shortened somewhat, and criteria for progression were more appropriate.

Shortly after its inception, the treatment model raised questions and curiosity in many people, since it was the first time, to our knowledge, that such a change had occurred. One of the curious people was Richard Russo, who ran the New Jersey Division of Drug Abuse Control. He assigned a New York State consultant to evaluate the program, and that person was impressed with the changes, though he knew of nowhere else using such a model.

I believe the LV phenomenon is still largely unknown, even by the professional community. I doubt it would be found, even in books and articles about TCs! Part of the reason is its short life. By 1973, Jersey City, New Jersey, used LV's three- million-dollar budget to build a methadone program, hastening its demise.

I moved to methadone programs elsewhere and also acted as a consultant to the NJ Division of Drug Abuse, evaluating and changing other TCs in New Jersey. An earlier reference to the "Zeitgeist" of Boring—the ghost in the atmosphere of thinking—occurred when I would visit a TC and the staff there had found the LV changes comfortable, anticipated, and justified.

Analysis Of The LV Experience

Though the LV experience may be interesting to read, my purpose is primarily to provide ideas about treatment to consider as we build a model of workable, testable theories and treatments.

Core Factors for Evaluation:
- Gender
- Race
- Power/control

- Outside-in/inside-out Treatment
- Personality Diagnoses

Gender was relevant because it was one example of "one size fits all." Women are not the same as men, but the common diagnosis of CD was primary—"A dope fiend is a dope fiend"—similar to AA's "An alcoholic is an alcoholic." The addiction *was* the issue, but we have known for many years now, and some knew then, that there were also other differences that mattered.

The TC staff were aware of some of this and, though they initially treated everyone similarly, they altered the program structurally afterward, with women's groups, to address the differences. Once again, however, the discussions there were dominated by the focus on addiction. Additionally, mostly all members of the hierarchy were male, so what message did this send to female residents?

Race was even more obvious, since the majority of residents were black at most times, with *some* black male representation in the staff. The message to women probably was: Men count and they have representation. The message to blacks probably was: White men count more.

Power/control was a background, partly unconscious, factor that drove LV's staff and resident behavior, as they drove irrational behavior in professionals on Tavistock weekends, and which they all were, by definition, unaware of.

In Tavy groups, the exercises were designed to elucidate the irrational aspects of human social and individual behavior. As a result, participants became more focused on interactions— the sources of power and its consequences.

Though we never did so, having TC staff attend Tavys would

have been very useful. It would have expanded their awareness and forced them to defend their views, in the process deciding whether to keep, modify, or discard them. Our transition required expediency, so we did the next best thing by choosing the more open-minded administrative non-residential staff, including business staff.

A key point in this discussion is the unconscious roots of power, as well as other behaviors, which had to be dealt with in a conscious, cognitive manner within the TC model promulgated in those days, as well as at present. The question is not whether this cognitive approach was the only modality, but whether it would have been changed if it could have been, and, additionally, whether the format would then have been more effective.

"Outside-In" vs. "Inside-Out"

The easiest procedure for TCs, and practitioners in mental health in general, is working from the outside in—imposing restraints and directing behavior. When deeper questions or "insights" are asked of the residents, they provided standard answers—the expected clichés to gain staff approval.

It is not easy for most people to gain insight, and it is very rare that practitioners in many areas of treatment have been psychoanalyzed or have even been in insight psychotherapy. The world has gone cognitive! It's far easier, more economical, and more testable. Whether it is superior, in the broad sense, is still to be evaluated, as I have attempted to do in later chapters.

In a more enhanced therapy being suggested, a practitioner would be involved with some form of insight therapy. This does not imply that residents would need to be treated in this manner, only that the staff would have a different view of the pathology, and operate differently, if they were treated in this manner—and thereby achieve different ends for their charges.

Chapter Eight

TYPES OF MINDS

BELIEVE THE CONVERSION PROCESS for LV would have been smoother if this had been the case. We are dealing here, as everywhere in life, with the human brain spectrum—from conservative to progressive.

The Conservative person believes that the past was a better time, and that all, or most, traditional ideas should be retained, not tossed aside for newer, less-tested ones. Progressives believe that the only constant is change, and that older ideas are to be exchanged for newer, more effective ones. Each has favorite stories that elucidate their point of view and reveal the folly of the other's.

In the TC culture, the conservative perspective in this example refers to the modality that saved their lives, not an academic debating point, so resistance to change is understandable and justifiable. However, justification of a position does not change the occasional *need* for change, and most certainly the *possibility* for change within that culture.

Resistance to this change means more; it is the resistance to almost *any* change. This degree of inflexibility filters down to residents and provides them with support for a set of ideas that may later threaten their sobriety. So outside-in approaches provide a level of encapsulation that achieves something at the cost of something else. The something else involves *substantive* changes (ideas, procedures) but not *process* changes (flexibility, power resolution).

To achieve this latter goal involves at least adopting an inside-out approach in some form, some insight therapy ideas and techniques to be added. This obverse direction means dealing then with unconscious areas of one's life, leading to resolution of inflexibility and power struggles that, in turn, lead to substantive changes in ideas and procedures, *not the other way around.*

Gender Issues

The last area—gender—is both a substantive and process one as anything else and, in this case, to address women's issues as well as men's, substantively, their representation in the TC hierarchy as expediters or group leaders; process-wise, it requires dealing with resolution of power struggles and inflexibility.

The ideas suggested here of enhancement of treatment are directed toward two ends. First, a TC could do more and needs to do more to resolve issues left relatively untouched. Second, that the deficits in TCs echo those of treatment elsewhere. These deficits will be addressed in later chapters, when theories and practice in academic and clinical psychology will be discussed.

Middle-Class Addicts

A relevant factor for any treatment approach in the early days was the arrival of mainly white, middle-class kids using serious drugs. Prior to this, older, browner, lower-class people dealt with their issues as did the ever-present upper-class people from perhaps several centuries past as well.

This change led to middle-class parents' pressure for different and more humane approaches to treatment and punishment. The "Zeitgeist" operated here as well as in the changes that took place at LV. Specifically, legal agencies lightened up, outpatient approaches proliferated, and chemical solutions were sought.

The chemical approaches had already been tried by traditionally trained mental health professionals such as medical doctors and, especially, psychiatrists. The meds employed were mainly tranquilizers (Librium/Valium)—to ease withdrawal, and anti-depressants (Elavil, Triavil, Wellbutrin)—to lift depression and make it a bit less likely that relapse would occur. Antabuse (Disulfram) already existed for instilling a revulsion to alcohol; its shortcoming was an alcoholic's non-compliance with daily ingestion.

The search for a chemical approach to treating opiate abuse/addiction was also underway. This drug, especially with IV administration of opiates by middle-class white kids, alarmed many parents. It led to the development of a substitute opiate originally developed in Nazi Germany in World War II and named Dolophine, after Adolf Hitler; it still exists today.

Methadone Maintenance

Dole and Nyswander, in 1967, developed a modified version of methadone at Rockefeller University that was made first into a wafer that was, later, replaced by colored fluids administered at methadone clinics; these clinics were originally funded by federal and state governments, which later provided that funding to private enterprises, as they do today.

At the time of methadone development, Richard Nixon was president and was enamored of the idea of using the drug to combat opiate addiction and decrease crime, primarily since opiates were of course illegal drugs. There was significant crime involved with heroin's procurement that occasionally led to physical abuse of innocent people, but mostly crime of the softer variety—breaking-and-enterings, robberies, and such. Further, it was manufactured in this country and required no foreign procurement.

Another aspect of crime occurred between addicts and their dealers. This type of crime differed from that today with cocaine, a stimulant, in which great violence occurs. The central difference is that coke is more expensive, and that the vast amounts of cash produced by its sale have enabled even very young people to become wealthy, and occasionally buy houses for their parents!

The possibility of dealers resolving their conflicts with their addict customers has been, and is, resolved by providing the addict with a "hotshot"—a much more powerful version of the drug they use, pure heroin for example, that leads to a quick death. Methadone alleviated all this tragedy if the addict wished it to; unfortunately, most addicts did not, nor do they now.

I believe we can view this use of a medication for addiction abstinence as serving, not primarily to help the addict, *but to alter criminal behavior.* President Nixon's administration was highly supportive of this role for methadone. It also was the first opiate replacement, as opposed to another "natural" opiate. It should in passing be noted that heroin does not occur in nature, but is chemically altered from opium, which does.

The original idea for methadone was to replace the heroin opiate with the laboratory-derived methadone opiate. Since withdrawal occurred when any opiate was terminated, it was thought best to maintain patients on methadone, called "methadone maintenance" (MM).

Methadone was more addictive than heroin, though it, like all other opiates, did not give the same heroin "high" that the two added acetyl groups gave to heroin. It did prevent withdrawal and thus satisfied the addict's cravings. This in turn allowed an addict to work and live a more normal life without crime—*if* they followed program guidelines.

MM clinics were and are open seven days per week because a patient requires daily availability to methadone when they are new to the program. After a social work interview for admission, the addict was provided with a physical, and any ancillary medical tests or evaluations; only then could a decision be made regarding program admittance.

The program consisted of MM only in the early days, followed by methadone detox, which was added for those never having been on MM, those under the age of eighteen, and those who did not wish to be maintained.

One must bear in mind that MM is essentially a legal addiction, only to a different opiate. Granted, the opiate did not give a "high" *if* the dose was only sufficient to prevent withdrawal and, more importantly, was under the control of professional nurses and doctors who limited the amount one could ingest.

So addicts had a right to be wary, and the federal guidelines respected this option by permitting detox(es). The end of the fourteen-day detox period resulted in zero mg. of methadone since the patient had tapered down from some modest dosage of 20–25 mg. The patient then had the opportunity to decide to leave treatment or increase their dosage to MM levels with a low of 40–50 mg. and, perhaps, a high of 75–100 mg. or greater.

It is instructive to note that, upon the inception of the MM program, guidelines had not yet been set for the maximum dose of methadone, so a large number of patients were on 200–300 mg. per day.

Take Homes

MM, as noted earlier, required daily doses, and this required daily trips to the MM clinic, which led to the provision of methadone bottles, called "take-homes," that allowed a compliant patient to provide the clinic with a locked metal box into which the bottles were placed; the nurse would observe the process of relocking.

The box was refrigerated to preserve the meth and, most importantly, to prevent others from ingesting it. If you or I had done so, respiratory issues would have arisen and, in some cases, death. In fact, there were tragic instances of infants and children dying in this way. Each bottle contained the exact daily dose required by the addict.

Take-home (TH) privileges were suspended if bottles were lost or diverted—sold or stolen. Neighboring MM clinics had different-colored liquids, so they could be traced to the dispensing clinic.

Another aspect of diversion was a patient not swallowing their dose and holding it in their mouth until they left the medication window, then spitting it into a container to be sold to another patient or a street-addicted person who couldn't get an opiate that day. It also was transferred into a waiting addict's mouth. To prevent this, nurses required patients to swallow and talk, as well as observing movement of a man's more obvious "Adam's apple."

If take-home privileges were lost, the patient then attended daily, or less frequently, if they had only part of their THs taken away. They would need to prove themselves with good behavior; a supply for vacations away from the clinic—sometimes across the country, or out of the country—were possible but suspect.

Non-Medical Phases

The detox and maintenance phases provided non-medical help in the form of a social worker (SW) whose job was to provide counseling. This counseling had to include the patient's dosage-change requests, bottle requests, vacations, life style, marriage, divorce, arrests, warrants, child support, debts, fines, and job changes. The SW would vote for or against the dosage change, and the clinical staff would make a decision confirming or denying the change, with final approval from the clinic physician.

The MM program was open-ended in time; a patient could stay as long as needed, even for a lifetime. This total availability of meds and staff is of course very helpful to struggling addicts but, as with any institution, comes to preserve itself as well. Making a profit for private and state-run clinics becomes a business in which profit can drive treatment.

MM Clinic Treatment Philosophy

A chemically driven treatment differs markedly from a drug-free facility like TCs. The goal in MM is to detox and maintain opiate abstinence for as long as possible *with methadone*. While some would argue that it also includes achieving abstinence, the possibility is very slim. Counseling street addicts, with their anti-social ways, is a challenge in any modality, and it is no different here.

In drug-free facilities, opiates were not universally given, and there was no protection needed for those drugs, as in MM clinics, where the draw is the drug. So manipulation wreaked havoc on protecting the supply. It was and is difficult for SWs to perform very effective counseling under these conditions.

Thus, the treatment philosophy was handmaiden to the chemical. The approach unwittingly promoted a lethargic state that militated against drug-free abstinence via detox from MM, as well as serious behavior change. This is especially true when so much effort is expended on managing the drug.

Opiates are not the only drugs MM patients use, all others are available to them outside and, unfortunately, sometimes inside the facility—cocaine, cannabis, barbiturates, stimulants, sedatives, and especially alcohol. Most opiate addicts/patients prefer other sedative drugs, though some use cocaine and other stimulants to reverse the sedative effect.

One of the major risks with this drug combination is an

opiate/coke user who drives or operates machinery. This involves the coke being metabolized faster, so that the user becomes very alert, with a subsequent rapid drop in stimulation when the coke wears off, with depressive retardation that could lead to an accident and death. This has also happened with opiates or other sedative-effect drugs like alcohol, barbiturates, and tranquilizers.

The issue in an MM clinic, then, is managing the opiate, and with urinalysis (UT) not being given *routinely*, even on a random basis, a patient can still be under the influence of another drug(s). The end result is a stable MM population that continues on its way with only the relatively cheap drug replacement for opiates. It is best for long-term addicts, who have little money and no insurance, to stabilize their lives.

In this respect, MM clinics provide a good service. However, in pursuing the historical threads of our discussion, MM treatment is almost totally chemically driven, and the patient is a passive participant. This raises the question—*why should one detox from MM?*

In my experience as a staff psychologist, clinical director, and outside consultant in MM clinics, I have seen many things. The power of an ever-present opiate in the bloodstream can block, not only cravings, but also pain. In fact, meth has been, and is, used for pain management.

In one clinic, a female patient had been maintained for years and then asked to be detoxed, which led to pain in her chest as the dosage dropped. X-rays showed a fulminating cancer she probably had for years while on MM, but the associated pain had not been felt until too late, and she died shortly afterward. She was on a high dose, and this situation probably has happened more often than we might think.

Another downside of meth is essentially being chronically addicted to a drug when other approaches are available. In the early days there was always drug-free treatment, though, in fairness, addicts tried these and failed; in fact MM was the last alternative for them, as they perceived it, and as it still is for some today.

However, today there are Subutex and Suboxone, the latter being the drug of choice for addicts because it can protect against diversion. Later chapters will explain this further. The downside of Suboxone is its cost. It would not only help switching MM patients to a different and more effective opiate, it would help those starting out before they could become MM patients.

Even more recently Naltrexone and injectable Vivitrol have been developed, the latter dealing with patient non-compliance.

The need for illustrating drug-free treatment in MM clinics is obviated by the inertia against it. The culture assists the drug in determining the approach, much as insurance company dollars have assisted briefer and, presumably, more efficacious treatment approaches while excluding others.

A second point is the power of a symptom-specific drug that replaces some or most aspects of drug-free treatment: withdrawal, anxiety, relapses, stability, self-confidence, etc. This *can* lead to a magnificent outcome but, as in TCs by their very nature, it diminishes the opportunity for other approaches. For the MM program to continue, drug-free counseling plays a minor role.

Is this, then, the same end point as in the AA or TC discussion—"We do *this* well, so others can do *that* well"? From one perspective, yes; but why do we permit partial treatments? It is not that MM patients are successful at even staying clean for very long periods, in most cases.

There are many CD people who are clean and sober but live lives of quiet desperation. Is abstinence our sole goal? Is it even our primary goal?

I believe abstinence should be our *initial* goal, since dealing with a person under the influence is not having a "patient" but an unguided missile. As noted earlier, a significantly enhanced program could be provided for a patient beyond their primary, secondary, or tertiary detox.

After a month or so in treatment, most of the negative effects of detox are over, and forward movement can occur—that is, of the internalized and memorialized variety. *It is at this point a balanced and complete program can begin the process of change more efficaciously than at earlier periods.*

It is also important for the initial program to offer variations of the treatment alternatives available. Even in the late 1960s and 1970s, there were central intake programs that directed people to a number of treatment choices—MM or detox, drug-free IP and OP, religious drug-free, private individual, drug-free psychotherapy, etc.

This is close to what I am suggesting but still encourages a specific single choice rather than, e.g., MM detox *followed by* drug-free IP, or MM detox and/or maintenance, *followed by* individual therapy. Of course, addicts can and do choose treatment alternatives themselves, but only after failures with their first or second choices, rather than holistically, from the beginning.

The risk of failure and relapse in between program trials can be very risky. If a central intake program monitored progress in each trial and received information about progress with the addict's approval, there might not be a relapse before program transfer.

The dilemma is not primarily the addict's predilections, it is the investment of the program in its own continuance, sometimes in opposition to the patient's long-term needs, that controls the process, since patient numbers determine funding.

Additionally, and surreptitiously, there is resistance between recovering addicts' inpatient and intensive outpatient program philosophies, versus that of chemical methadone treatment programs.

It is worth noting that a treatment person or professional cannot ethically choose for others what might be best on a subjective basis. It is at this juncture that analysis of one's mind would alter this bias—justified by the *moral choice of saving others*—as such people prefer to see it.

A carefully thought-through discussion will lead us to one dictum: *There is no single way to reach abstinence.* This dilemma of the unexamined mind will follow our discussion, as well as the biased persons' lives, always.

Chapter Nine

CHEMICAL SOLUTIONS OVER THE DECADES

The '50s

NITIALLY, TRANQUILIZERS (Valium, Librium), anti-depressants (Imipramine, marketed as Tofranil, as well as other tricyclics—known as such for their three-ring chemical structure), sedatives, hypnotics, and Antabuse (Disulfram), were used to quell the angst of addicts and alcoholics. Antabuse would lead to involuntary expulsion of stomach contents if alcohol were ingested. Unfortunately, its efficacy was ameliorated by non-compliance—the alcoholic not taking the pill daily.

Agonists and Antagonists

Agonists are a class of drugs that act upon receptors in such a way as to mimic the effect of a natural drug, e.g., methadone.

Antagonists are a class of drugs that oppose the effects of drugs, e.g., Naltrexone, which occupies receptors—in this example opiates—and "blocks" opiates from occupying those same receptors.

The 1980s—Antagonists

Narcan, an opiate antagonist, later marketed as Naltrexone, was used in the early '80s to deal with life-threatening overdoses of opiates and induced comas, in emergency rooms (ERs).

Buprenorphine was introduced in 1982 in the U.K. It was later sold as Suboxone and Subutex. Initially, it was a pill held sublingually; in recent years, it has become available as a film for quicker dissolution and to lessen its bad taste.

Subutex is pure Buprenorphine and is used for those patients who are not at risk for diversion (selling or passing on the drug).

Suboxone is composed of two drugs—buprenorphine and naloxone. Naloxone's role is to place the patient into withdrawal if they ingest an opiate.

This phenomenon can be dangerous to the uninitiated sychiatrist or physician: A psychiatrist with no addiction experience, who also did not know what the term "bricks" of opiates meant, prescribed Suboxone for a patient that led to inpatient hospitalization.

The 1990s

Campral (Acamprosate Calcium) was first introduced in Europe and was employed, as an adjunct to other medications, to stop the alcoholic from drinking. Its action was unknown, but it was able to "balance the brain," i.e., to mediate the ill effects of alcohol withdrawal.

In my experience with addiction psychiatrists, it was a short-term phenomenon, primarily, I think, because of Naltrexone's ability to occupy the same overlap of receptors related to opiates and alcohol, but in a more effective manner.

The Millennium

Naltrexone has continued its great success in a new form—a liquid injection called Vivitrol that is provided IM in one's gluteus maximus or butt.

The greatest advantage to any injectable is its ability to completely control a patient's urge to use for at least three weeks to a month. Non-compliance of addicts with oral medications is probably legion, and Vivitrol was a welcome addition to the opiate treatment arsenal. It is the most effective chemical treatment I've seen in fifty years.

Chapter Ten

STATE-OF-THE-ART TREATMENT PRINCIPLES

DSM-V And Acting-Out Personality Types

THE DSM INDICATES SUCH ACTING-OUT TYPES as Impulsive, ADHD, and Anti-Social, with impulsivity being present in others as well. This nosology is, of course, a pathological one and offers little help with how such individuals' minds work from other, normal, perspectives.

Psychological Differentiation: Internalizers and Externalizers

This concept is quite old and well established in the psychological literature and has a Gestalt orientation. The book *Psychological Differentiation* (Witkin, Karp, & Goodenough, 1962) via experimentation reveals the concept of a scale of learning/living styles, on a spectrum from Internalizing to Externalizing.

The authors found those on the Externalizing end learned from the "outside," being more responsive to external cues and having difficulty incorporating, storing, and implementing information. By comparison, Internalizers employed outside cues as well but could easily assimilate information, as well as organize it, internally. The concept of types of structure within the brain purportedly directs this process.

This general difference is not only evident in learning, which is its broader and more interesting aspect, but also Internalizers and Externalizers respond differently to emotion and sicknesses. An analogue to understanding the differences superficially is that Internalizers are more like obsessive-compulsives, and Externalizers are more like Impulsives, somewhat like ADD types.

The evidence that patterns which control behaviors are genetically driven occurs here as well. The notion that many behaviors we see are *only* learned is simplistic; that they are *primarily* learned is more arguable, but only in certain behavioral repertoires. The balance of genetic vs. learned proportions varies with behavior/brain types and, of course, with our state of scientific knowledge as well.

ADD-Definitions, Diagnosis, Treatment

ADD and impulsivity can be viewed as part of the externalizing dimension. The "outside in" assimilation indicates the genetic basis for such behaviors and a way toward formulation of treatment regimens. It seems futile to continually reinvent theories for explanation and treatment when those that exist are useful and sufficient.

The biological bases take priority—"Ontogeny recapitulates Phylogeny" is mainly true. Psychological/psychiatric assessments precede the administration of medicines and are followed by treatment with effective and relevant therapies.

In the case of ADD, for example, there is a need to rule out several other diagnoses: Asperger's, mania, depression, anxiety, and learning disorders. Learning disorders are not the same as ADD, which is technically not a learning disorder, though it certainly has a powerful effect on learning.

The best routine, time-saving psychiatric or psychological assessment, is the DSM-V criteria effectively administered. Employing a written version of the ADD criteria from the DSM-V prevents rash decisions to rule ADD in or out.

Subsequently, a stimulant, or a non-stimulant like Strattera, might be given. A trial of either type of medication in a diagnostically confusing patient could easily settle the problem. The typical psychiatric regimen is to prescribe a stimulant medication because it acts much more quickly and provides an earlier decision about whether a patient is ADD.

As we know, ADD is not learned, it is inherited. The environment plays its usual role of channeling, but genetics run the show and drive symptoms. If medications are not used, especially in moderate to severe cases, therapy is likely to be defeated or at least made more difficult.

My advice is to use medications, even in mild cases, because the inability to attend, concentrate, remember, and organize is the quintessential "learning disorder." I have never understood the resistance of professionals to categorize ADD as such, but no matter its name, it will interfere with life and psychotherapy.

In any event, with regard to the CD population, ADD reportedly occurs 10 to 15 percent of the time. In my experience, the rate of occurrence is far greater. The difference is explainable in part by the accuracy of assessment. This, in turn, varies according to who does the diagnosing—internists, pediatricians, psychiatrists, psychologists, social workers, counselors—and how.

Recovery and Risk of Relapse

Recovery requires that many areas of a CD person's life be structured. The closer the program/therapist is identified with AA and behaviorist philosophy, the more singular the focus on abstinence. This makes sense, especially if the therapist is recovering themselves, and, more to the point, we tend to repeat what we have been taught and what has worked for us. The difficulty with such "true believers" is their greater resistance to changing, or even elaborating upon, their point of view.

It is clear that abstinence is primary, but of course activities of daily living are also, as noted in LV's experiences discussed in earlier chapters. It is sufficient to briefly mention relationships, vocations, hobbies, finances, legal issues, etc. Beyond A.D.L. (Activities of Daily Living), there is the long past which affects the present and controls it.

The focus here is on recovery and relapse. The general program headings, as above, could be transposed to any comprehensive therapeutic program, but the view of human behavior and the techniques employed to achieve change would differ.

Aside from the therapeutic approach presented in this book, there is the critical and central aspect of controls versus freedom and the notion of permitting acting out, and even designing it into the program.

Specifically, does a program require strict controls on

freedom/acting out, or more lenient ones? It is true that the type of personality being dealt with is most important, but the issue being raised here is different from that.

Does one allow the freedom to act, or even to act out, under a broader more flexible set of controls in early to mid-recovery, to permit the "relapse" (drug or behavioral) to occur in milder form followed by the possibility of remediation? I believe the answer is yes.

It is the *perception* of relapse that is important. If a CD patient perceives relapse as a heavily anxiety-laden act, then relapse urges will be fearful, guilt-driven events. When the relapse does occur, self-recrimination will reign, and the likelihood of another relapse is unwittingly reinforced.

The challenge is to deprive the relapse or urge of its emotional power by approaches such as relaxation and opposing urges experienced in and out of therapeutic sessions. There is a parallel in this approach with analytic ones.

The Calm Scene of Robert Benson's relaxation approach (*The Relaxation Response*, 1975) is one of many possible and effective techniques. The patient is asked to recall a place they have experienced in their life that makes them feel more relaxed than anywhere else. The patient then closes their eyes, unfolds their arms and legs, and focuses only on the calm scene.

It achieves its best results with exacerbated stimuli that are actually in the calm scene they have experienced. For example, if the scene is on a beach, the sea gulls, waves, heat, sand texture, smells, and sounds are all incorporated to recreate the real event.

When intrusions occur, patients are advised to not become anxious or attempt to push the intruding thought aside, but merely to say, "Oh, well," to themselves, and allow the thought to slide away "like water off a duck's back."

An additional issue is a patient who already employs meditation/relaxation. They can either employ the Calm Scene or continue to employ their own, provided their own is intended for relaxation and not for goal setting or some other activity.

This approach can be extended to Systematic Desensitization, a behaviorist approach (Wolpe, 1958) in which a list of anxiety-arousing events/people is hierarchically listed from least to most arousing. The least arousing are experienced first, then the more arousing, and on up the list.

Role of E.M.D.R.

A different approach is progressive relaxation—the tightening and relaxing of muscles from one section of the body to another, accompanied by deep breathing. The approach I use requires about 30 minutes and exists on numerous CDs (e.g., McKay & Fanning, 1986)

During training for E.M.D.R., we were taught a color relaxation approach that involved the patient's imagining a colored ball on top of their head. The color needs to be one the patient finds relaxing. I usually use blue, because it has been chosen by many patients.

The words used by the therapist are also spoken at a very slow pace. This point cannot be emphasized enough, since pace is significant in producing the state of relaxation, so much so that normally paced speaking can greatly reduce the relaxation state; think of listening to a speech. Slowly spoken words slow down the patient's thinking and thus their feelings.

To continue, the blue color gradually moves from the blue ball to the patient's skull, where it cools down and slows the brain's activity, then proceeds throughout the body from top to bottom. The process takes about eight minutes and works extremely well.

There are of course many relaxation procedures that can be matched with the therapist's and patient's desires. The major point is, some form of relaxation is critical with impulsive, pressured people so they can "hear" your message and keep their demons at bay.

Chapter Eleven

CLINICAL INTERVIEWS
ACROSS THE PROFESSIONS

The Mental Health Traditional Model

Clinical Interview

Mental health practitioners existed prior to AA, and it is reasonable they would treat CD people as though they were neurotics or character disorders who just happened to be using chemicals. Since psychoanalysis ruled the day at that time, some CD people were analyzed.

In hindsight, there were many difficulties with that approach:

- An exploratory approach pursued UCS causation. The problem was lack of awareness of the addiction process and the assumption that abuse/dependence was mostly beyond one's ability to control.
- Such practitioners were not accustomed to patients proficient at disingenuousness in using drugs/alcohol, denial, in coming high to sessions, in assenting to behaviors to become

good, to compliant patients, as well as to "doctor shopping" for prescriptions.

· The general trend of lying on a couch required someone who could attend and focus well for insight purposes; CD patients, however, had significant cognitive impairment at the initiation point and for some time after they achieved abstinence.

· The practitioners assumed that CD patients were intelligent and as insightful as the average expectable analytic ones they knew.

· They also assumed that CD patients were inclined to peruse their minds for insights as their demons harassed them.

· Most important of all, they further assumed that any inability to improve was the result of "resistance."

Given the analytic paradigm, gathering information and making inferences from it was defeated from the start. Mental health dynamics of any type, not just analytic ones, could not account for biochemical bases of an addiction process. Even AA's philosophical assumption that alcoholism was inherited did not and could not make this assumption with the knowledge base in effect at the time.

The closest parallel for the persistence of addiction was O.C.D. (Obsessive Compulsive Disorder), which mental health professionals were familiar with. However, even though OCD looked like addiction, the theory presumed psychodynamics as an explanation and not biochemical addiction.

Interlude

In subsequent years, from analytic to later Rogerian therapy, there were parallel developments—traditional treatment and assessment on the one hand, and non-professional recovering people on the other.

To their credit, recovering people and AA supporters were correct in deciding traditional approaches didn't accomplish much as they took risks with a CD person's life. In this situation, trying something else, and especially something that resonated with their own experiences of recovery, seemed eminently sensible.

That new recovering/AA approach was a seat-of-the-pants operation that achieved some important goals. It would be a few decades, until the 1970s or so, before recovering people would be provided with professional training and some academic knowledge.

The State of New Jersey, and others, established "schools" for training recovering and straight (non-recovering) treatment personnel. This academic idea was very important in the process of raising the level of discourse and therapy, because it employed professionals and made them consistent; I was one of those professionals.

The Recovering Chemically Dependent Model

The recovering person is typically someone who has a varied level of education from no high school to a master's degree, with or without chemical-dependence training for alcohol or drugs from a professional school. As in all these characterizations, I am speaking of the "average expectable" individual, a term employed by psychoanalyst Heinz Hartmann.

Clinical Interview

There are similarities among such individuals, such as the anxiety and dysthymia as part of their addicted past, still present, along with probable genetic family histories. Additionally, the means of their having achieved abstinence is relevant. AA/NA recovering people have a more truncated view of what works and what doesn't, primarily because one tends to become wedded to what helped them achieve abstinence.

Therapy with professionally trained CD mental health-based personnel is usually seen as less effective, perhaps because the early personnel in the field did not know more than mental health dynamics and viewed addiction as primarily "mental," and therefore a matter of "will" and sometimes, "morals."

Consequently, such individuals may view themselves as superior because they can "identify and relate" to the CD person. While this is true, and AA/NA has worked well for many CD people, there are other approaches—many paths to the same goal of sobriety.

In my experience, the recovering person's mind is narrower, concrete, and definite about what they believe. Their style is reminiscent of defensiveness in someone who feels less secure and somewhat diminished about their lesser role in treatment teams.

Sometimes this leads to an isolationist view that contends, "We know more about how to end addiction—our process has been around longer." I have seen TV ads that now state, "We deal with the deeper aspects of addiction." It should be clear by this point there is a great deal to the "deeper issues" that is unknown to most of these practitioners. We might regard such language as "marketing."

Given this background, openness and flexibility are mostly absent. Thus, for them the "correct" approach is easy to administer, all the more so if the recovering professional has achieved sobriety via a specific path. In most cases, if the patient/client resists, this professional emphasizes their greater knowledge and that they have already done what the patient is attempting. It often becomes a child–parent paradigm.

The clinical interview is merely a matter of obtaining the standard bio-psycho-social information. In this regard, information is controlled by the format required. However, as in treatment, there is a difference in the amount and quality of what is obtained.

If one is neutral and inquisitive, then information flows more naturally. If one prejudges the patient and views them and their answers as right or wrong, the interviewer will be consciously or unconsciously forcing the individual into a mold. This view applies to any professional or inquirer.

The general nature of the interview process is more authoritarian when interviewers know what you know and may be intent on proving their greater knowledge and experience.

Thus, they are more reliant upon their judgment and experience in interviewing.

It could be argued that the lack of formal assessment tests, albeit even with the use of the DSM-V, reinforces reliance on one's subjectivity and allows a counselor to maintain their interviewing stance as well as the correctness of their views.

Objective tools challenge our assumptions. By this I do not mean that subjectivity has no place, only that it is too unrevealing in and of itself. Intuition plays a significant role if expressed by experienced and/or sensitive people.

Mental Health CD Specialist Model

Clinical Interview

These professionals include all manner of practitioners, including psychiatrists, psychologists, social workers, and counseling professionals. In many respects there are some differences among them, but there are many similarities as well regarding the clinical interview and the administration of CD inventories.

Psychiatric Model

As most people know, psychiatrists are trained in the assessment and treatment of abnormal human behavior. Psychiatrists, physician's assistants, and psychiatric nurses are the only medically trained mental health personnel, and the only ones who may prescribe medications are psychiatrists and P.A.'s.

Clinical Interview

The central issue here is the means of assessment. It is a clinical, essentially non-test, approach as carried out by other mental health personnel with regard to the bio-psycho-social information.

One difference is the emphasis on medical history-taking and trenchant diagnostic evaluation via the DSM. Although other personnel can use the DSM, they ordinarily do not have the same skill level as psychiatrists, who developed and maintain it, and if there is a difference of opinion among personnel, psychiatrists' opinions hold sway.

In spite of the sophistication of DSM terminology, the issue of ADD diagnosis noted in an earlier chapter is germane. To have criteria and not employ them stringently is a problem in CD treatment and elsewhere. The price for diagnostic miscues is maladaptive, or less than optimal, functioning, including relapses.

Based on my observation of addiction and psychiatrists' approaches, their first step is to obtain mood control, assuming psychosis is not also present. Then, once that is achieved, they attempt to deal with secondary, or co-occurring, diagnoses, e.g., character disorders (AXIS II), ADD, learning disorders, etc. In my opinion, the major contributor after mood and character disorder, for addicts, is ADD.

I have heard a minority of psychiatrists state that ADD plays a minimal dysfunctional role in adults. However, this does not appear to be true, for at least two reasons. If ADD, and more specifically ADHD, is present in adults, it was present earlier in life, because it is inherited. Also, without some level of control in those years, that individual was more prone to acting-out and less able to attend and concentrate, and therefore do well in academic subjects, as well as in their daily life.

So the propensity for maladaptiveness is present and provides a platform for abuse or addiction. Because of this central role for ADD, it becomes a priority to medicate, in some or most instances.

Medical Labs

Medication's role in CD treatment is the same as in other contexts—primarily to stabilize the patient, so psychotherapy can take hold. In the case of ADD, it is much more difficult, and unnecessarily so, to treat without it.

No matter the choice of psychotherapy—analytic to behavioral to dynamic—all depend on attention. Incidentally, the eyes averted/closed approach described in a later chapter, including lying down, allows greater focusing for everyone, especially the ADD patient, because it diminishes intrusions.

The psychiatrist's role is primary, in my view, because of the power of present-day medications. An even greater role is described in the next chapter, which considers how the psychiatrist and psychotherapist collaborate regularly to modify patient behavior to an even greater degree than medications alone.

The specific steps for diagnosis in psychiatry could be detailed for a number of conditions, but I have chosen to elucidate ADD from the DSM, which has this list of characteristics describing the triad of inattention–hyperactivity–impulsivity.

The questions focus on early life behavior, since ADD is inherited and would be most obvious then. Asking for the present-day functioning level for each item is also necessary, in my view, to determine the present symptom picture.

The issues involved in the diagnosis of ADD reveal the sophistication of the psychiatric approach to diagnosis as well as the folly of using its criteria as a simple check-off list, of which psychiatrists are well aware. While evaluating whether the patient has any of the criteria, a need also exists to rule out other diagnoses that mimic ADD: anxiety, depression, mania, learning disorders, and Asperger's, for example.

To negate the rule-outs is part and parcel of the complete psychiatric evaluation for this syndrome. Navigating the criteria for ADD can be a stumbling block. Most psychiatrists enunciate the criteria by asking the patient whether he or she has any of them, but also make their own interpretation from the patient's behavior, sometimes regardless of the patient's protestations to the contrary.

I believe that, some of the time, ADD is missed in part because practitioners don't use a sheet such as the one from the DSM-V, and also because they don't elaborate upon each characteristic. Additionally, the sheet can be used for interviewing the patient's significant others separately, or together, and comparing answers.

Secondly, whether the diagnostic process is embellished by use of a DSM sheet or not, the number of items to reach criteria—6— may not be reached, but does this rule out the presence of ADD? What if there were a 5 or 4? We must remember these numbers assigned to lists were not scientifically derived.

From an evaluative perspective, the assumption that the absolute number 6 has more validity and reliability is possible, in large part, because the degree of thoroughness of the evaluator limits the exactitude of the score. Given these weaknesses, we would be unable to assume this state of affairs.

I have worked with psychiatrists who agreed to a medication trial even with a lesser number of items. Ordinarily, the initial process involves the use of a stimulant as opposed to Strattera, the only non-stimulant ADD medication, because it will show change in days rather than weeks.

Finally, if there is a disagreement between practitioners, there is no loss in a trial—if the patient improves, they probably have ADD; if not, they probably do not. This point cannot be emphasized enough; the great contribution of ADD to maladaptiveness, especially in CD patients, demands its careful evaluation.

Social Workers/Counselors

In my experience, social workers and counselors have the most social and conversational approaches to assessment. Each tends to believe their primary task is to understand their patient's/client's issues through inquiry into their family and present situation.

The core of their beliefs, in general, is very likely to rely much less, or not at all, on genetics and the belief in pre-ordained behaviors as causative. As time passes, this has also been changing because of the increasingly accepted role of genetics.

The treatment approach is similar: that the therapist can change things by talking almost exclusively, with little or no reliance on the other leg of a more complete treatment approach—medications.

The general penchant of these professionals, in my experience, has been that, even in cases of suicidal ideation, there is a reluctance, sometimes, to refer for medications. In one respect, this style reinforces the power of the therapist, which can attenuate the rate of change and thereby enhance risks. As to historical information gathering, the bio-psycho-social format should be a minimum.

Psychological Model

These professionals are the only ones licensed and capable of administering psychological tests. I am leaving aside those situations in which some non-psychologists are given special permission by test manufacturers to use tests in studies or research. In daily practice, psychologists have tests available to more objectively assess a patient's functioning, not just their intellectual aspects.

It will require a lengthy discussion to tease out the elements of this important argument, because there is a tendency to see all evaluators as being more similar in the validity and reliability of their assessments than they are or can be.

Objectivity—Measures of Validity

Clinical Interview

The discussion of objectivity is not, "It's more objective because we say so, and besides, it looks that way." In fact there are seven types of validity in test assessment: face, construct (criterion, convergent, discriminant), generalizability, standardization.

Face validity is precisely that: "It looks like it." It is the simplest type and states the obvious; e.g., if a test claims to measure auto mechanical ability, we expect it to have questions or statements about cars, engines, transmissions, etc.

Construct validity is the most essential of all and asks the question, "Does this test measure what it purports to measure?" Construct validity, in turn, subsumes three types of validity:

- Criterion:

    Concurrent—Does the test measure the same construct as other tests that are similar?

    Predictive—Does the test predict an individual's performance in specific ability areas?

- Convergent:

    Self-report scores on other tests

    Trained interviewer ratings measured against self-report scores

- Discriminant—Essentially that the test doesn't measure what it isn't meant to measure, that it discriminates. There should be a low correlation (r) between test A and test B, because they are measuring different things.

- Generalizability—So far in our presentation, a test may be valid according to the above measures, but are the results of test A equivalent to those of test B? Additionally, a test may be valid and reliable but not be generalizable to another, similar measure, or to other populations besides the one from which the norms were drawn.

- Standardization—Tests are considered to be standardized when they are administered under similar conditions, are scored objectively, and are able to measure relative performances, i.e., performance relative to the normative group, and not to the test taker's class or reference group.

Testing—Computer-Scored Personality Measures

A psychological examiner has the capacity to measure mood states like depression with surveys, like other professionals, but can add the BDI-II (Beck Depression Inventory). Personality can be assessed by the Millon Personal Inventory (Pearson Publishing), 16 PF (Personality Factors—IPAT, Champaign, Illinois), or PEPQ (Psych Eval Personality Questionnaire), MMPI, etc. In truth, there are tens of thousands of psychological tests in existence (Buros Mental Measurements Yearbook, 2017).

Intelligence Testing

Intelligence measures are legion, but the Wechsler series of intelligence tests is the most highly regarded, and for good reason. It should be noted that IQs obtained through these tests, which can only be administered by a psychologist, are the most valid, reliable, and complete ones available to the field. All other intelligence tests—essentially group-administered ones—have validity and reliability based upon the Wechslers (WPPSI-IV, WISC-IV, WAIS-IV).

The Wechslers have additional advantages over other IQ tests. To know someone's IQ, no matter how valid and reliable it may be, is not terribly useful. Wechsler developed his tests to go beyond the early Stanford-Binet IQ test, which had a single IQ score and was highly verbally loaded.

Wechsler wished to measure both verbal and performance aspects of intelligence as well as adding a combined full scale IQ. The WAIS, for example, has 11 subtests to measure verbal and performance intelligence: six for verbal, and five for performance, as follows.

VERBAL	PERFORMANCE
Information	Picture Completion
Digit Span	Picture Arrangement
Vocabulary	Block Design
Arithmetic	Object Assembly
Comprehension	Digit Symbol
Similarities	

The validity and reliability of this test are not dependent on the assumptions of those unaware of test construction and statistics. Though the subtests above may not look like they can measure intelligence, they in fact do; that is, they measure what has been defined as intelligence by psychologists—as someone has quite correctly noted, "Intelligence is what intelligence tests measure."

An intelligence test probably measures one's *capacity* to learn—the higher the IQ, the better the learner. Another view is that it measures the *speed* of learning.

The central issue is the common agreement that this measure is the standard. The following examples of WAIS subtests will not include specifics of their test content because that is not permitted by ethical guidelines.

So the WAIS measures intelligence and does so by tapping into a great variety of behavior samples that, by themselves, provide significant reliable information about someone, even from a psychiatric perspective.

For example, to know results of the Comprehension subtest alone can give the reviewer information about language level, intelligence, emotional appropriateness, and psychosis, for starters.

When one considers the totality of verbal subtests, the results are more robust. *Information* taps general information about the world and is not merely a limited measure of one's acquired academic knowledge. If there is a significant deviation in this score from other scores and the full-scale score, it might point to deficits or self-education, for example.

Digit Span measures one's ability to recall a series of numbers forward and backward, and this reflects the test taker's level of attention and concentration, mostly the former. It is possible to see intrusions, with reference to psychiatric functioning.

Vocabulary taps the subject's knowledge of words and, in turn, indicates the level of overall intelligence, because this test correlates .85 with it. If this score is diminished, it may indicate a loss of a formerly higher level of functioning, and this may, for example, be the result of injury, infection, mental illness, chemical toxicity, or retardation. Conversely, a proportionately higher score may mean self-education and/or advanced education.

Arithmetic does involve basic math processes in word problems. The ability tapped here is a measure of attention and concentration, mostly the latter. As noted earlier, Comprehension provides a measure of social judgment and appropriateness.

Similarities offers the manner in which one word is similar in meaning to another—from concrete to abstract aspects. As such, it reflects thinking on the concrete/abstract dimension— important for a psychiatric diagnosis.

Raw scores—the absolute number of correct items—are converted to standard scores, a relative value based upon the normal curve, enabling comparisons. Significant deviation from the average value has relevance for level of functioning from intellectual and emotional/psychiatric perspectives.

In summary, the WAIS has properties for assessing intelligence and emotional (psychiatric) functioning. It should be noted that content or thematic analysis, not a formal part of the WAIS at all, is available to any examiner with such knowledge.

This approach comes mainly from the field of psychoanalysis, and was incorporated into Rorschach testing first, followed by other psychological tests, and it is most ably represented by the works of psychoanalyst and psychologist Roy Schafer (*Psychoanalytic Interpretation in Rorschach Testing*, 1954).

Schafer employed thematic analysis with the Rorschach and applied this approach to the Wechsler tests, as has also been done with the Thematic Analysis Test (T.A.T.) and any projective test. This adds a dimension of assessment that psychiatrists especially would employ if they were psychologists.

Words, and their associated affect, are the key to unlocking the mind's mysteries, no matter which test or assessment instrument you choose. Let us not exchange higher-tech approaches derived by science for that dating back to the beginning of spoken communication—language and its meaning, the first assessment.

The Verbal subtests are only half of the intelligence domain measured in the WAIS but indicate the sophisticated level of assessment available to the examiner. The other half of the WAIS subtests are the Performance ones:

Picture Completion: The subject views cards with simple line figures and determines which parts are missing. Because the drawings are simple one could make the case that many parts are missing, so the direction is, "Yes, but tell me, which parts are missing?" This test taps judgment and social insight, leading to a measure of the patient's level of appropriateness.

Picture Arrangement: Composed of a set of single cards with drawings like those in newspaper comic sections. The goal for the test taker is to ascertain what the whole story represents and then to rearrange the card order to represent the best story they can tell. The test permits alternate versions of the story as well. This requires the ability to anticipate social events and their outcomes and can point out paranoid tendencies.

Block Design: Employs small blocks with variations of color on all sides. The examiner presents the blocks and points out the different sides and colors. He/she lays out the blocks in a design format, then asks the subject to match the designs' colors only on the top of the blocks. After a few administrations the examiner presents the design on cards to be copied. The test requires eye-hand coordination having bearing on neurological function as well, involving part/whole concrete/abstract aspects.

Object Assembly: A puzzle with large parts which require the subject to ascertain the whole, then produce what is noted. Again, this involves part-whole and concrete/ abstract aspects.

Digit Symbol: A transfer task which is timed in which the subject observes a series of numbers and matching symbols, then uses this series to write in symbols below the numbers. This task requires correct observation and speeded functioning.

I cannot provide more information than I have to a non-psychological audience because of restrictions on sharing data that is copyrighted, but mainly to avoid revealing it to those who might one day be intelligence test subjects.

The central issue in this phase of the discussion is to point out the objectivity and sophistication of assessments psychologists can employ. This permits something no other evaluator can claim--that the raw test data obtained by one psychologist can be interpreted more correspondingly and completely (inter-rater agreement) by a second psychologist without the latter ever having seen the subject/patient; this is a powerful tool.

The lack of structural objectivity in other clinical evaluations does not permit this. Psychological tests from other evaluators, e.g., MMPI, are not up to the task and, most importantly, are usually completed by computer, so they are not "raw."

Attempts to use the MMPI raw data leads to a less broad and accurate evaluation than those of psychologists, even though the MMPI was developed along the lines of psychological tests and mostly by psychologists.

I realize many will counter with the observation that other fields have the capacity for blind analyses, and that these have been performed for many years. The difference I am alluding to, however, is the term "structural objectivity" noted above.

Although it is true that most fields of inquiry can perform such an approach, the level of accuracy is dependent on the level of objectivity and mathematical representation possible--reaching its apex in psychological tests.

Chapter Twelve

THE RULER: NOMINAL, ORDINAL, INTERVAL, AND RATIO ASPECTS

THIS ARGUMENT INVOLVES THE EXPOSITION of levels of experimental inquiry as nominal, ordinal, interval, and ratio scales. This system of organization was developed by Stevens (1946, 1951). As brilliant as this idea is, it has its critics: Rozeboom (1966) and Michel (1986).

The scales were developed to categorize data types, so they might be evaluated by differing statistics. The purpose was to make psychology comparable in measurement with a general science's approach.

- *Nominal* refers to just naming things
- *Ordinal* refers to rank ordering things without having fixed distances between the items: positions on a scale—1 to 10, so 3 is lower than 5, and 5 is lower than 9. This scale allows relative differences but not precise distances between those numbers in this case.
- *Interval* refers to a scale with precise distances, for example,

on a temperature scale, 49 degrees is 2 points above 47 degrees, as 97 degrees is 2 points below 99 degrees.

• *Ratio* refers to a scale with an absolute zero with no assigned value, so the differences are precise and measurable; but in this case there is the possibility of multiplying values and stating, "This point is twice the value, or one-half the value, of X." So the ratio is composed of all the aspects of nominal, ordinal, and interval scales besides containing its own characteristics of ratio capacity.

Briefly, non-psychological inquiries are at the nominal/ordinal level, but psychological tests like the WAIS are at the interval level.

Scientific inquiry is mostly at the ratio level. Essentially, the field of psychology is more scientific than other non-medical fields and psychiatry, when one does not include medical lab tests.

Of course, lab tests can provide physiological/biochemical information that has some reference to psychiatric inquiry, but no serious investigator/practitioner would regard them as mental assessments—merely as corollaries anticipating neurobiological approaches.

The latest approach involves genetic aspects and their relationship to medications (Genomind-genomind.com)

A sample patient's report can be found on that site. The company is one that does genetic testing and projects results for appropriate medications from that protocol.

The headings from the report compare Gene Results with Therapeutic Implications, Interaction, and Clinical Impact. Additional information is provided primarily for categories of medications. My major reason for including Genomind is to present psychiatry's future in the present, and its physiological evidence for dealing with treatment issues to advance the DSM as well as psychiatric treatment.

My closing thoughts are on marking off some number of inches. Such a device possesses all the aspects of Stevens' system.

A ruler has names for inches, spaces between the numbers, fixed intervals between the numbers, and the numbers can be added, subtracted, multiplied, or divided and have an absolute zero. The ruler, in this regard, is superior to the mental health systems we have discussed!

A Different View of Treatment

Approaches to alter behavior:
· Medications alone
· Psychological—cognitive/behavioral therapy
· Psychoanalytic therapy
· Other therapies

The combined model considers "specific path to access change," which views "ancillary" aspects of psych factors as "primary" in the process of accessing change, regardless of the particular school of therapy practiced.

For example, ADD is not "something else," but the first step on the path to accessing the mind, and therefore primary to the major psychological presenting issue of, say, addiction or other acting-out. (It is not primary for detox, only for post-detox issues.)

ADD Model

ADD meds, particularly Strattera, improve attention/concentration to access the mind for change in affect, anxiety, impulsivity, and poor judgment—all of which prompt behaviors antithetical to positive change. Any of these can especially interfere with insight-type therapies.

Thought/Mood Model

Medications for clarity and greater appropriateness of thought/affect lead to clearing away the usual debris that hampers a more realistic and measured view of reality by the patient.

CD Model

Alcohol use leads to diminishing affect and interpersonal in-volvement with "ownership" in relationships, including with the therapist. "Ownership" is the ego participating in a full and active manner, not just while under the influence.

Abstinence without medications would lead one to believe the mind is clear and free of obstacles, but secondary and tertiary detox are a real biological phenomenon and, in turn, affect the ego—the CS (Conscious) primarily, the partner in change. It is not necessary to entertain the contribution of UCS (Unconscious) aspects of func-tioning here, but they are relevant and will be addressed later.

Medications that are helpful—some would say necessary—in treatment include:

- Vivitrol (IM injection) or Naltrexone (pills) for maintaining abstinence from alcohol/opiates
- ADD meds—stimulant and non-stimulant types
- Anti-depressants
- Medications for borderline thinking/psychosis like Abilify and, more recently, Latuda.

The basis for this cadre of medications is that the syndrome of dynamics in a recovering alcoholic typically involves ADD and depression. Borderline/psychotic symptoms occur somewhat less frequently, but in my experience, more frequently than they do in the general population.

In some estimates, including my own, this syndrome, minus borderline aspects, occurs in the vast majority of alcoholics. Finding it is a direct function of one's diagnostic skill; essentially, as always, "If you don't see it, you can't treat it."

The central issue is not whether the syndrome exists; many, perhaps most, practitioners agree that it does. That issue is the need to address all symptoms that are present with medications, to make the process smoother to traverse as a first consideration. Oftentimes, there is little or no progress without medications—a problem for verbal therapy-only therapists.

The second, and related, aspect is the role medications play in access, again that the syndrome is primary, especially in early recovery, not a set of symptoms to also be addressed as they present problems later—a critical difference.

Incidentally, when practitioners do not see such issues early on, they of course don't recommend medications or even address the issue itself. However, even when they do observe these issues, the syndrome is typically viewed first, and perhaps singularly, as a manifestation of "resistance" or "denial."

Related to this is the sophistication of the practitioner's knowledge of, and openness toward, medicine and medical practitioners.

Many practitioners come from fields of treatment that preclude and even demonize such approaches. This occurs partly because medicine and its practitioners have not had a very sterling track record in the past, and partly because avoiding medications is "natural" and empowering to the patient and perhaps, unfortunately, to the esteem of the therapist.

Treatment, and its relationship to medications, varies primarily with relation to the practitioner's personal biases/skills, not only what they learned as tenets of a formal school, or schools, of therapy. This set of therapist dynamics requires confrontation by the therapist, or their supervisor/therapist, to resolve personal issues.

However, even after the therapist accepts this approach and the necessity to address previously described ancillary aspects as primary, there are still obstacles.

Specifically, there are other levels to this approach involving fine-tuning of medication types and dosages in response to the level and type of dynamics in therapy at a given point, not to prescribe them as a generally stable dose during therapy.

Take as a simple illustrative case an individual who has ADD and is provided with meds—e.g., Strattera and an SSRI— as well as therapy. Medications diminish ADD symptoms, so therapy can proceed to deeper levels that otherwise would have been stymied by inattention and inability to concentrate.

As therapy proceeds, or as life presents stressors, however, anxiety and inattention are worsened, and medications need adjustment. As before, this adjustment should follow therapeutic need and not always target general relief of symptoms. The goal is to maintain the patient on a course of maximal participation in therapy.

The approach sounds typical so far, but it probably isn't. The likely view of the therapist, when ADD and anxiety features "reappear," is that they will probably be accepted as a "resistance" issue. This notion harkens back to psychoanalysts in the past—and some in the present—who disparage and discourage medications as blocks to therapeutic progress. Essentially, they believe that patients don't experience the full level of anxiety attached to the traumatic event, and that reduction of it by medications cheats patients of the opportunity for empowerment via insight. It would be more difficult, however, to make this case for ADD meds, since attention and concentration are necessary—for psychoanalytic insight especially.

PHARMACOLOGY

The study of chemicals and their effects on the brain represents the basis of what we see from a behavioral "psychological" approach.

The effects can occur in other parts of the body, but the brain is the area we will focus upon primarily. Drugs must become water or fat soluble in the body in order to cross the cell membrane and thereby have their intended effect(s). For our purposes, THC ("pot") is the only fat-soluble drug—all others are water-soluble.

Alcohol

Alcohol is the most popular and easily obtained drug, and it is viewed by most people as more benign than any other. It is worth noting that alcohol reputedly has been used by those with more educated and cultured life styles, and that it has been available legally for most of its history.

This probably began with "captains of industry" who popularized the notion. It has been noted that the fermentation process for making alcohol was discovered by Arabs, but there is evidence of dried ethanol in some 9,000-year-old pottery (ethanol history.com).

Alcohol use moved from Middle Eastern countries to Europe and the rest of the world. Its value was, and is, related to its sedating and depressive effect. This aspect made alcohol popular as a "social lubricant" for those with difficulty socializing. If anxiety is decreased, it allows users to say and do those things not easily accomplished without it (Fillmore, 2003, p. 179).

Alcohol also acts to disinhibit by depressing the areas of the brain that inhibit our daily actions. In this way we feel more open to engage in activities that are difficult or not possible at other times.

Genetic aspects

As with all drugs and other behaviors, there is a genetic component to alcohol use. This sets the stage for inherited tendencies that begin the process of becoming a non-user, user, abuser, or dependent person.

This initiation process does not determine the trajectory of abuse and dependence, but does aid in their development. Environmental aspects control the rest—family, financial, emotional, and social stressors, and diet, in the main.

Ingestion of Alcohol

Alcohol is primarily drunk and processed in the stomach, liver, kidneys, and intestines, where it enters the blood stream. There is a "solid state" ingestion of alcohol, which was popular in the '80s and '90s primarily among adolescents—"Jell-O" cubes. Alcohol is added to a mixture of gelatin and allowed to cool to a solid.

When solid, it is ingested and eaten, thereby entering the stomach in a state that allows slower assimilation of the gelatin and the alcohol. The great danger of this is the greater sudden release of alcohol in this tasty food that allows the body to be overwhelmed with more alcohol than if drunk, and some users have died.

Alcohol's Effect on the Brain

Alcohol and other drugs then travel to neuronal receptors and, when present, they release chemical hormones—neurotransmitters—that produce the behavioral effects we see and feel when under the influence.

For example, the chemical serotonin can lead to relaxation and sedation, and dopamine to a bright mood. Until the alcohol is metabolized in the major organs of the body and in the receptors, the brain is under this influence. When the receptors are emptied of alcohol, a hangover results from the withdrawal.

At this point the receptors want more alcohol, and the user accommodates their desire, often believing they are "making" the decision. In truth, their brain generates the need through the withdrawal state and the accompanying mood and behavior unpleasantness.

As we can see, the action phase of the process is at the receptor level, and science has created medicines that can block the receptor sites that drugs occupy. When this occurs, the drug(s) in question cannot produce their usual effect until the medicine occupying the receptor sites is metabolized, requiring the drug's ingestion and the beginning of habitual use, given the presence of other factors.

Medicines for Alcohol Treatment

Medicines used for alcohol treatment in recent years are:

- Antabuse (Disulfram), an old medicine in use since the 1950s that induces nausea and vomiting when alcohol is used while on Antabuse. The shortcoming of this medicine is that an alcoholic can avoid taking the oral pill the day he or she wishes to drink, without negative effects. Antabuse is not a chemical "blocking" agent.

- Narcan (Naloxone) is an injectable or inhalable medicine that induces sudden and thorough withdrawal from opiates. It was introduced in the 1980s and saved many addicts' lives. The process involves its reaching neuronal receptors and "wiping away" the opiate occupying those areas. The sudden withdrawal leads to agitation, and sometimes anger in the addict because of a sudden loss of the pleasurable state.

- Campral (Acamprosate) is a blocking agent that reduces cravings during withdrawal and held promise as an adjunct for Naltrexone that could reduce cravings prior to use. At the time, such thinking was worthwhile, but, with Vivitrol eliminating this aspect of Campral by reducing craving reduction in the first place, and on a continuing basis, things changed.

- Vivitrol—(an injectable form of Naltrexone). The advantage of this more expensive form of Naltrexone is its effectiveness especially in treating medically non-compliant patients. Vivitrol is always present and does not rely on a patient's memory or desire to use the medicine. Once it is injected IM, the CD patient cannot undo its effect for 3 to 4 weeks, depending on the particular person's metabolism and use history.

Campral has rarely been used in recent years, while Antabuse is still used in some quarters. Overall, Naltrexone and Vivitrol—the same medicine—are the preferred approach used today by most addiction MDs. A thorough listing and explanation of medications to treat alcohol exists in Johnson and Ait-Daoud (1999).

Opiates

Natural

- Opium
- Morphine
- Codeine

Synthetic

- Dilaudid
- Demerol
- Oxycodone
- Vicodin
- Fentanyl
- Methadone
- Heroin

Semi-Synthetic

- Oxymorphone (contains thebaine)
- Hydrocone (contains codeine)
- Oxycodone(contains thebaine)
- Hydromorphone (contains morphine)

The Quick Detox

This "treatment" is no treatment at all. It consists of employing Narcan, which wipes the opiate receptors clean of opiates no matter how they were introduced into the body. In the past decade or so, there have and continue to be physicians who provide this approach mainly, in my opinion, to those financially well-off individuals who abuse opiates during the week and then check into a hospital.

There they are anesthetized, and Narcan IV introduced. After an overnight stay, they leave feeling normal to begin their week or more at work before being hospitalized again.

As one can see, this approach has no beneficial long-term effect, since it only enables the addict to continue using without experiencing the usual side effects for very long. As such, it is not like any other treatment. I only mention it as, thankfully, a generally fading approach in the long history of CD methods.

E.M.D.R.

The above issue also relates to E.M.D.R., as one competing example, in which the traumatic event is aroused, and then a distraction of a visual/auditory/tactile nature is provided by the practitioner's device, to rob the trauma of its anxiety-arousing value, thereby effecting therapeutic change—even without insight. It should be noted however, that post-affect reduction, rational aspects of thought, and insight do occur.

Such a possibility, and actuality, challenges the psychoanalytic postulate of "no gain without pain" by increasing reduction. Besides that, it also supports the view of outside manipulation of internal mind events to allow the patient to control external events, achieve empowerment, and proceed to still deeper issues. The substantive difference is what is done with the new material.

The notion presented so far of a partnership between the therapist and medical practitioner—preferably an addiction psychiatrist—and the use of medications, is common.

What is uncommon is the idea that assiduous and effective use of medications can allow change in therapy not attainable through other approaches—even those that use standard medications—but outside the framework of this interactive approach.

Such an approach leads to greater behavior change, in both degree and type, as a result of this view of "secondary" symptoms as primary. They have a role in therapy as behaviors are diminished over time and then replaced by a more effective life adjustment.

Patient Readiness And Protocols

It is widely stated that "You can't help someone who doesn't want to be helped." Although this seems to make sense, it may not be so. If someone is resistant to treatment, there are many options left to convince or force him or her. This is not what I recommend, but all options must be considered, no matter how impractical, when the situation is dire.

1. Family interventions are useful, if performed with the help and participation of a professional. The confrontation involves members in an alliance with each other for the good of the patient, and it may include pressures from guilt, insistence, and discussions about future contingencies: "You can't live here anymore, we will not provide you with money, you will lose your S.O., etc."

2. The legal system—when a patient is arrested, the court's involvement is often extremely helpful by demanding treatment or jail. Often, families are encouraged to not aid their child with monetary or legal help to avoid the court's sentence when this occurs. I had a patient whose father called the police when his son left to obtain drugs on the street; the father even drove him there. This led to an arrest and probation. The probation officer demanded continuance of treatment or else, and this led to his "cooperation."

3. Persuasive aspects of therapy—the CD person wants certain ends, and the judicious use of medicine and verbal agreements help. For example, a CD person, virtually always, self-medicates; even seeking the "high" is self-medicating, since this state helps to obliterate the pain of their lives. Offering psychiatric medication that can deal with patient symptoms is similar to self-medication with street drugs. If a patient is anxious, SSRIs help to ameliorate this; confused and inappropriate thinking is resolved with anti-psychotics, etc., to provide alternatives to street drugs. Approximating the medications used illegally is the most acceptable alternative for CD patients. Of course, the replacement medication is not identical, but it is closest and seems preferable to abstinence. Medication is defined in some quarters as "a drug is a drug."

4. Use of the therapeutic alliance. Therapists can ally themselves with the patient to assist with the family or the courts, in exchange for useful cooperation with behavior change.

Therapeutic Patient Positions

The traditional psychotherapeutic position is patient and therapist sitting in chairs opposite each other. The traditional analytic psychotherapy position is a patient lying down, with an analyst seated behind his or her head. Lying down has certain advantages—relaxation, avoidance of eye contact, and improved ability to concentrate and facilitate free association.

Patients are not required to lie down in this approach, since the key aspect is avoidance of a direct visual angle. The prone position helps addicts who can't stare into a therapist's eyes, often because they like refractory angles for manipulative purposes, as well as those who have ADD or other syndromes that inhibit openness and concentration.

Resolution can be achieved in alternate ways:

- Patient sitting and therapist turning his or her swivel chair around
- Patient sitting and closing his or her eyes, as in relaxation approaches. In fact, relaxation approaches can be helpful in their own right with this approach.

One of the advantages of this arrangement is reduction of anxiety—sitting up increases or maintains anxiety and avoidance; a prone position decreases anxiety and can therefore diminish defensiveness and increase openness and acceptance.

There are some individuals who experience paranoia, but there is an adjustment for them, too. It is useful for the therapist to turn their chair with their back to the patient. This gives the patient control of most everything.

Besides patient position, of course, medications aid change. The central goal of medications, in my view, is to change the brain to ameliorate basic issues for therapy to become effective. Essentially, psychotic individuals become more reality oriented, acting-out types become more controllable, and mood-disordered ones become more stable.

Adding a more effective insight approach yields a three-part plan composed of position, medications, and verbal technique that is, at least for the present, state of the art.

Insight Techniques

Before expanding on the couch or eyes-averted approaches, I must add that it is difficult to find even analysts who use couches— they mostly employ face-to-face positions, like the cognitivists who have mostly replaced them. The major difficulty with this is the inability for a patient to associate as freely to their inner life.

If one considers making eye contact with a therapist who stares back, it is clear that very little useful reflection occurs. Conversations that replace therapeutic inquiry are not analytic, or particularly helpful, endeavors.

Use of an eyes-averted approach is the commonality in any system of therapy that is recommended here. Beyond that, the first major hurdle, and the one that takes many weeks or months to achieve, is forgoing rational thought for emotional pursuit.

When someone first participates in this manner, they typically have a hard time avoiding thinking about and reporting information as if they were in standard face-to-face therapy or counseling. Patients believe it is safer and easier to continue in this way. However, this results in therapist and patient remaining near the surface of dynamics and events in the patient's life.

If one observes what occurs in standard therapy, patients routinely report the past week's happenings; to drop this is not easy, but drop it they must, to engage the approach I propose. Analogs include explaining they will need to follow feelings to other feelings, and then to related ideas. To surrender oneself to this is a lot like keeping oneself at the threshold of pre-sleep when one feels drowsy and is about to surrender to unconsciousness.

If it is not forthcoming, the therapist can withhold their own verbiage until the patient is proceeding in the manner indicated. Not speaking is consonant with this approach, the reverse of face-to-face counseling.

The task for the patient is to relax, so insights are approached through emotional connections rather than intellectual ones, then to understand the connections and incorporate them in their lives. Only the first stage differs from cognitive/behavioral approaches and it is most important because it is more effective.

To make conscious connections, or "insights" or "behaviors" or whatever your lexicon, is not useful to anyone, especially the patient. One could make a connection for someone, or lead him or her to it, *and the resultant "aha!" moment is impressive but usually leads to little change unless the patient recalls it at the critical, teachable, emotionally expressive moment.*

Consider the example of a patient, who was referred for anger management, experiencing no significant change in knowing his behavior was related to earlier life experiences. Only after an interpretation was made by the therapist connecting the patient's emotional state that was being acted out in the session, was the patient led to his surprise and insight.

The less surprising the interpretation's acceptance, the less valuable it is likely to be. The "surprise" indicates the patient's unconscious information has been revealed and the connection made.

Subsequent to this, he no longer was able to respond with hostility to such events. The difference between cognitive insight and emotional insight is quite significant, even if the cognitive therapist employs what seems like a similar approach. The technique helps if therapists use an eyes-averted arrangement, use much less verbiage, write effective notes, and, most importantly, have been analyzed themselves. These days, psychoanalysis is passé because of its perceived weak heuristic value and great expense.

–

Chapter Thirteen

THE TAVISTOCK EXPERIENCE

N MY EARLIER CHAPTER ON THE LIBERTY VILLAGE therapeutic community, I mentioned Tavistock as the experience the staff undertook during the transition in treatment modality. I had first attended a "Tavy" weekend during an earlier phase of my psychoanalytic psychotherapy at Columbia, and as an adjunctive modality. (A professional explanation of Tavy groups can be found in Shapiro, Edward, & Carr, 2012, pp. 70-80).

Tavys differ from other group experiences, like "T" groups, in the same way analytic approaches differ from cognitive/ behavioral ones—much less emphasis is placed on conscious processes and heavier emphasis on unconscious ones. The shift also induces emotional regression.

The system is based on psychoanalysis but mainly focuses on social systems rather than individual ones we might customarily expect, and with specific focus on the expression of "power and authority." Theorists who developed ideas upon which Tavys drew include Melanie Klein (1960), Wilford Bion (1959), and Boris Astrachan (1970).

The processes were developed at the Tavistock Clinic in London, then exported to other parts of the world, particularly the U.S., and particularly at Yale and Columbia. I attended the weekend at the City University while on the faculty of the New York Medical College, then later with the L.V. staff.

The group of professionals who provided the Tavy experience were from the Institute for the Applied Study of Social Systems (I.A.S.O.S.S.) in both instances.

At the first evening's meeting with Tavy staff and weekend participants, the "leader" explained the "contract" to all of us. Essentially it included the purposes of the experience:

- To explore power and authority in groups
- To delineate the role of the "consultants," who were not called "group leaders."
- To explain that the consultants would meet with us in assigned rooms, and that we had a schedule of the weekend's activities. The assignments separated friends and acquaintances.
- The groups would be separate, as well as observed by other group members—the "fish bowl" technique.
- The consultants would not only "run" our groups, there were extra consultants who would have their own group, to which we could gain entrance during the weekend. The purpose would be to observe their group in action.
- At designated points during the weekend, all consultants and participants would meet in the large room.

We did not understand how serious the initial explanation of the contract was regarding our roles in the process. If we had, we would have listened more intently and asked more questions, since they meant every word. We only realized this later, during the large-room combined meetings, where we and the consultants clarified those terms and processes.

The first group required us to meet in the assigned room at 7:30 PM on Friday, though many of us arrived earlier. Precisely at 7:30, the consultant arrived, sat in the empty chair, and stared at the floor. At first we awaited the "leader's" description of what we should do. He not only demurred on this account but never introduced himself or even addressed anyone.

After we realized we were on our own, we introduced ourselves and told a bit about our jobs and careers. Then we fell silent, searching for another topic. As we did, the group's anger surfaced and was directed toward the consultant, who was deemed rude and asocial. Some of us told him so, and then he responded, but only commenting upon the group's behavior, not any individual's.

It was clear that, no matter how seminal an individual's comment might be, it would lead to nothing from him. In this instance, his comment addressed our anger and that it might be related to the group's anxiety. This led to even greater anger, because he not only refused to participate in ways we deemed appropriate but then criticized our opinions.

He told us nothing about himself, and we gradually adjusted to the role he played and the roles we were left to play, with the burgeoning realization that we were responsible for our behavior.

However, besides owning it, as other non-Tavy group experiences also taught, we had the dual level of conscious, and psycho-analytically interpreted unconscious levels of our experiences to internalize as well.

Related to this is our reactions to the regression induced in the groups. We were all mental health people—psychiatrists, psychologists, social workers, etc.—and on one evening, some of us wanted to throw the consultants out the window; others found the electrical box with breakers and threw the switches to cut power everywhere.

This was 1972, and only recently, in 2016, at a major psychoanalytic society meeting, I queried a speaker who was psychoanalyzed, but with unresolved issues, who stated he had attended a Tavy but had been "frightened."

During the "fish bowl," when we observed others, we noted they were similar to us. We also saw the consultants' group and noted we could not gain entrance as easily as we had assumed, because they had a person come to the door they called a "gatekeeper." That person asked us our business and then closed the door to address the consultants and explain our request. If they chose not to see us, he told us so and closed the door again.

This simple process of controlling us so the group could proceed with its business, then acting quickly and decisively in dispatching us, made us feel power-less and power-full at the same time. It made clear the use of power and authority, as they promised. All observations in such groups, including non-Tavy types that are successful, hopefully teach lessons we keep for life.

The additional point I would like to make, however, is that Tavy groups made me and others aware that the effective and legitimate use of power led to different personal and professional behaviors and outcomes. This difference occurred in work with patients as well, of course.

As an example, when most therapists take a position on a patient's behavior, they are often unsure and choose to avoid pushing their and their patient's authority to the fullest, for the benefit of both. Each must realize not only that all options exist and, further, are to be owned by each, but more importantly, that greater health and functionality require this.

So if a person states they cannot oppose their lover, for example, the question is why. The discovered answer is some version of "It would be hurtful to one of us," and then to "My past prevents me." The role of the therapist, in my view, is to suggest the pursuit of more directive and power-full behavior. The end result may still be that they don't do it, but the mind has been stretched to include the previously unthinkable as possible.

I do not think it is easy for the therapist or patient to fully understand this difference without the corresponding emotional charge and change that drives all behavior, and one obtainable in part via Tavys. For those who have not internalized this difference, a patient or therapist may be seen as cool and calculating rather than actualizing and empathetic.

It should be noted the consultants were employed by L.V., not only to provide the weekend Tavy for others and ourselves, but to visit L.V. and meet with key administrative staff. To illustrate this approach, the consultants who visited us and obtained information, then returned to a single consultant who never visited us, and who listened to their story for distortions and manipulations. So the consultants themselves accounted for their own defensive behaviors with another level of interpretive safeguards.

Tavy Influence on Therapies

Power and authority are germane to all human behavior, including therapy, regardless of one's theoretical orientation. So what did we learn from this Tavy exercise?

The central benefit, in my view, is its focus on power and authority outside the confines of a particular theory, even though it has been derived from a variant of psychoanalytic theory. Experiencing a Tavy weekend does not expose one to much psychoanalytic interpretation, though it is true that psychoanalytic interpretation does exist in the literature and practice outside Tavy exercises.

 Rather, watching oneself act out unconscious drives provides the primary evidence for one to understand and internalize, regardless of one's favorite theory. My experience, as well as that of others, is that having another dimension of oneself opened up surprises most of us.

Additionally, there is the issue of changing one's approach in therapy, and life in general, to dealing with boundaries to control behavior—yours and your patient's. Many therapists are too lax with times for appointments, makeup sessions, availability for questions outside the session, billing issues, taking phone calls during sessions, dealing with intrusions from the waiting room, etc.

The above issues are variations of transference– countertransference, defined in part by boundary relationships in Tavy language. Boundary problems can be partially avoided from the start by composing a policy that makes boundaries clear, along with their attendant resolutions.

However, the major aspect involves one's awareness of problems and their resolution. It is easy to make the case for an insight approach, especially a psychoanalytic one, in this regard.

The examples above are practical matters, but theoretical and therapeutic ones are more salient. How does one account for the primitive and unconscious drives that therapists have never addressed in themselves?

Additionally, how does your acting-out during Tavy exercises change your view of patient acting-out? It no longer allows acceptance of the more superficial emotional states you saw before yours were uncloaked. "Reality is in the eye of the beholder."

Once you see this, do you make changes in future patient assessments, or in how you deal with emotional states? One specific change post-Tavy is the legitimate, effective, and persistent use of power and authority in ways that non-Tavy therapists view as bold and overdone, even inappropriate. This seems to occur because they are not aware of *their* UCS issues.

Priorities In Early Treatment

The first step in treatment of an active CD person is the same as it is with non-CD ones: to establish rapport. CD people present the additional issue, alluded to in the opening chapter, of mistrust. This is especially true of those with co-occurring disorders, perhaps with confusion and distortion added as well.

In traditional Mental Health (MH) populations, even today, such personnel are viewed as helpers. With CD populations, it is reversed, and there are several levels to the discussion:

1. The usual MH dynamic of rapport establishment between

two strangers leading to a treatment alliance
2. The physical action of chemicals on the brain in altering reality contact makes for amenability
3. The mental imbalance of co-occurring disorders
4. The CD "street culture" of mistrust, in the case of street addicts

The process of establishing rapport and the treatment alliance does not begin in the treatment office—it begins with the person making the referral. It is necessary to coach the referral source regarding aspects of therapist competence in CD, and the nature of the therapist as a person.

Therapeutic competence is, hopefully, a given, but information about the therapist as a person may be less so. The central reason is its value in fostering patient comfort and acceptance. CD people generally have poor self-images, and this leads to great resistance to therapeutic personnel, whom they perceive as being too well integrated in comparison to themselves.

There is threat value in this, which can be diminished by familiarity. In fact, the therapist as recovering addict is most comfortable of all—"You were like me, so you know." Conversely, "You're no better, you were an addict, too!" which provides him or her with protection against potential debasement and a built-in basis for defense later, when confrontation occurs.

Therapeutic Flexibility

The ability of the therapist to tolerate change and challenge in patients is vital. Therapist rigidity evidences a need to control, therapist flexibility evidences allowing and cooperating with others in the process of change.

Some issues are:

1. Modeling a behavior that CD people don't typically possess—open-mindedness. Their ability to change, sometimes quickly, is not open-mindedness but a lack of intellectual and emotional involvement in the principle at issue. In other words, from a therapeutic perspective, opinions that don't mean much are not useful as a means for system change.

2. An ability to tolerate stress associated with maintaining a contrary point of view from theirs, and not responding defensively with emotions or ideas.

3. An ability to change opinions with ease, if the evidence warrants it. Related to this is not changing simply because of pressure—theirs or that of others—but as the result of evidence and reasonableness alone. They must see this difference, namely the change that results in a change in the system structure, not the specific content change of an idea alone.

4. That, if no one changes their opinion, people can still continue to relate without conflict, by just "agreeing to disagree."

Should a therapist be unable to model this behavior, the CD system ends up maintaining more than just one rigidly held opinion—there is instead a systemic refusal to adapt to the process of change, a very important omission for a teachable moment on the way to eventual permanent behavior change.

The Matrix Outline

It is easier and more effective to construct a diagram of the ongoing information about, and dynamics of, the patient from session to session rather than collecting and rereading copious notes. This diagram is related to a genogram in representing issues and relationships spatially.

A sample matrix follows:

Initial session

I.P.: 19-year-old male John heroin dependent—6 yr. history—failed at IOP and IP Tx-searching for "cure," possible Vivitrol, non-compliant. Parents terminated relationship—no CD history in family—no arrest history.

S.O.: Mary, 18-year-old enabler, non-user-R (relationship) of 6 months—4 prior relationships of 3 months or less.

Plan: Vivitrol primary or Neurontin.

Session 2

S.O.: more controlling than thought, not only enabling but provoking re: her need for attention and money

I.P.: willing to steal more for her—too much risk for arrest—referral made to psychiatrist Dr. O.—EMDR begun.

The outline format saves many words, is easier to read and reread, spaces permit later changes without rewriting, and there is more time for treatment, etc.

Chapter Fourteen

ISSUES IN INDIVIDUAL THERAPY

THINK IT WAS HERE—it never was there," says Pippin, in the play of the same name, realizing his ideas were an illusion for his continuing development.

The initial contact and the therapeutic alliance has been addressed earlier, with particular emphasis on differences between CD and non-CD populations.

Honesty

The CD patient plays fast and loose with the truth because he is engaged in duplicity to obtain chemicals, while simultaneously hiding the truth about this aspect of his life. As such, the therapist needs to maintain an open but jaundiced eye toward any reporting.

Assessment

This does not mean the suspicious approach employed by the average expectable law-enforcement person, but a healthy balance of what is best described by a modification of Erik Erikson's term "triple bookkeeping." This involves culture, individual style, and genetics (Erikson, 1953).

Every one of us is composed of genetically controlled matter set within a given culture and mediated by differential response sets to environmental interactions.

It is important, in ascertaining genetic contributions, to employ a four-generation genogram. In this way we can have extensive and thorough information about one's past. This offers a broader schema of an individual's predilections than any practitioner's investigation and intuition can obtain in as short a period of time.

The CD person who has behaved with a fair degree of integration will be viewed differently if we know that a first-degree relative had a virulent form of CD or a major psychiatric disorder.

Establishing probabilities at each phase of treatment is essential for thoroughness. The Matrix spatial representation of patient information is a very helpful, if not necessary, technique in this regard.

Knowing the CD patient's culture, formal and CD-related, adds to our understanding of the degree to which they would likely act. Their interpersonal relationships provide information about response tendencies at any given time; these changing tendencies can be represented in the Matrix system and their implications reassessed over time.

If a CD patient still has drug-fulfilling connections, or works in a high-risk career, or engages in self-defeating behaviors such as dating individuals who have proven destructive to them, then we have a better idea of what is likely to come.

Employing this triple bookkeeping approach provides the therapist with a more effective way to assess information given at any time in the relationship with their patient. The major advantage is its avoidance of frequent and direct confrontations, which can have a deleterious effect on the therapeutic alliance—even while the patient in early treatment may still be engaging in duplicity.

It seems counterintuitive but it is also true: One must treat a patient in the manner we expect them to behave while they still behave in ways we do not sanction, and they are not as yet in accord with where we ostensibly hope they will move.

Resistance

This behavior is treated no differently from dishonesty. It is more effective to employ a refractory, rather than direct, style in confronting resistance, again because it leads to less patient resistance. This should not be a competition for autonomy; it should be an opportunity for development of internal commitment and cooperation from the patient.

The CD patient is always struggling with autonomy with everyone, including his or her therapist. To deprive them of a sense of security is to only increase their resistance to adopt your offer of a different way to deal with life. To persist in controlling them is an issue of yours they need not deal with—and another reminder of the necessity of a therapist's own issue resolution.

I am not suggesting patients should not be confronted, especially when situations demand it, only that, when possible, the confrontations be *in*-clusive rather than *ex*-clusive. This "partnering" on the long journey of life's changes is essential.

Splitting

The therapeutic alliance is most threatened when this occurs— the CD patient's playing of one person or professional against another. The issue is probably best handled by a straightforward recitation of the need for honesty in all relationships, especially those with the therapeutic team—physician, family members, etc.

This is best reinforced by your modeling of these principles in your own therapeutic and personal life because you always know more about yourself.

When confrontations occur with regard to "splitting," you must not, however, revel in the superiority of your moral high ground; rather, state the situation in neutral terms as a rule of the process necessary for patient progress.

Timeliness

CD patients are often notorious for lateness and forgetting—a first-rate reason for changing the brain with medications, in this case treating any ADD issues, for example. Once one is satisfied that such psychiatric diagnoses have been accounted for, timeliness is represented as one more boundary-breaking behavior.

One must realize that boundary breaking is "testing" the therapist and attempting to control treatment. For the therapist to relent by not addressing it is to diminish the alliance—which is not to be confused with the therapist trying to enforce control for its own sake, perhaps a neurotic issue of the therapist.

It is most useful to represent the difficulty in patient, or other, terms thereby reinforcing boundary relationships. The patient must know at least two aspects of the problem: that their lateness could impinge on someone arriving after their scheduled time. Also, therapists should not delay the succeeding patient's session start, though other professionals such as organic physicians might.

More importantly, it is valuable to describe lateness as patients cheating themselves of treatment time. "I am mostly concerned about not having the full amount of time I have allotted for you." In such a patient's view, shortening the session time via lateness is a strategy to shorten contact and get what only what the patient wants, though the therapist has professional needs as well.

At first blush, it appears this is only a cognitive issue to be dealt with cognitively, but, as always, it can be more than that. The deeper basis for lateness may be reflective of past relationships with authority figures for example, and as such have another level.

Chapter Fifteen

ISSUES IN GROUP THERAPY

Modeling

G ROUP DYNAMICS ARE PARALLEL to individual ones in an interesting manner. In individual therapy, the therapist withholds interpretations and suggestions until the patient has an opportunity to internalize the insight or behavior. In group therapy, the therapist remains one step behind this process and allows group members to internalize and offer insights and behaviors to each other first.

Remember, the overriding goal is, of course, developing patient autonomy. The group merely adds another level for the therapist in allowing other patients to be "therapists" first.

It is true that patients do and probably should model themselves after their therapist's more efficacious behaviors; however, this modeling should not be mimicry—for example, saying the same phrases or employing their mannerisms.

Rather, it is best if "process" aspects are internalized, as in adopting delay in reactions or responses, empathizing with others, and revealing personal motivations for therapeutic purposes. It is hoped that this is balanced by being a group member and responding from that perspective as well.

Splitting

Of course, therapists would monitor "patient as therapist" behavior. One disruptive aspect of misdirected modeling is a patient playing the therapist role as a means of separating himself or herself from others. This behavior is one of the most deleterious in individual or group therapy because it shifts the balance of power and control, with at least two effects:

1. Shifting legitimate authority from the therapist, whose role is to facilitate everyone.

2. Allowing the patient to diminish his or her benefit from the group. This "insulation" from treatment harkens back to the T.C. discussion in the role of the "expediter."

Timeliness

A cautionary note before this discussion is begun. By "lateness" and "absence," I mean repetitive infractions, not occasional, excusable ones.

Lateness differs in group, as opposed to individual therapy of course, since it is multiplied by more than one patient. In individual therapy, the late patient delays the start of only his or her session. In a group, one or more individuals don't delay the start; in fact, all but one being late won't either.

Starting the group with one member is acceptable, but—and this is very important—it is not necessary, or recommended, that the therapist only allow the one group member to speak about himself or herself because the other members are late or absent.

This prohibition is widespread in therapeutic communities and in recovering groups in general. I disagree, because it allows dissonant members to hold the group process hostage. Additionally, without a "price" to be paid, late and absent members learn little about their responsibility to others. In any event, the absent member can be filled in later, if the others or the therapist wishes so.

Fraternizing

This issue, again, has a parallel with individual therapy. Patients meet each other in the waiting room and often, legitimately, come to know and like each other, which can lead to socializing outside the group.

This behavior may be acceptable in many areas of life, but it isn't in therapy, and it must be effectively confronted. It is a special case of "splitting," in separating the therapist from his or her patients.

Absences

The acceptable number of absences depends on the total number of sessions. If the group runs longer than a few months, then one absence per month is about right. In a standard group of 1.5 hours, a lot is covered that is difficult to make up.

The major basis for controlling absences is, as always, to emphasize the culture, the serious basis for meeting, the people chosen for their interest in the group. Additionally, in my practice, group is additional to individual, so any one who wishes to drop out could still continue with individual treatment.

Alfred A. Borrelli

Therapies As "Tools"

It has become customary to tell professionals in training and conferences that they are about to learn another, new approach that becomes one more "tool in your toolbox." To name an approach a tool is to reveal the cognitive categorization of treatment; more importantly, *you* are the tool.

The problems with this are conscious application and the confusing assumption that different therapies can be combined, even if they are not all cognitive.

This may be a good place to mention that psychoanalysis is not employed to deal with the training analyst's mental disturbance—there may be little or none. The purpose of psychoanalysis is to reveal and resolve, especially, unconscious issues that would interfere with analysis of an analysand.

In fact, there are two types of analysis for preparation: individual analysis first, followed by a training analysis to evaluate and remediate issues that might arise between the analyst and analysand.

Coursework in an analytic institute concurrently completes the training. It is relatively common for an analyst to return to analysis—perhaps with his or her training analyst when analyzable issues arise. As one can see, this career is a most- of-a-lifetime investment. On its face, it is clear this is very different from all other mental health training.

A Therapeutic Approach

The difference between CBT and an analytic analogue is most evident in UCS aspects, but additionally in therapeutic engagement.

| 216 |

What I am about to elucidate is similar to an analytic technique, but somewhat different.

It is necessary for non-behavioral therapists to connect to patients on emotional and thought bases, including perhaps the "observing ego." The "observing ego" is an analytic term for that process which allows us to observe simultaneously, not only the patient, but our own assessments of that patient, as we proceed.

The process I am suggesting is a match between therapist and patient, in which the emotional and thought connection is coupled with the observing ego in such a manner that the therapist is parallel to the patient's processes. The difference lies in the activeness of the connection.

In essence the therapist, in a metaphor, is not observing the patient's roller coaster ride from the ground, but is in the car with the patient—observing while participating.

In an analytic approach, there is observation, and recording of and responding to, information. In this approach the connection is such that the patient is aware of the therapist's presence and influenced by it.

The influence is not the type that directs the patient's judgments, but provides them with a perceived "other" that promotes a review of the issue at hand, essentially a self-examination.

The value of "eyes averted" or "lying down" to this enhancement of the examination of one's consciousness should be clearer yet. Further, the practitioner's successful personal analysis is central to allowing the non-judgmental posture to be actualized with much more success and be less tempted to blame it rather than himself or herself.

Chapter Sixteen

THEORETICAL CONSTRUCTS
AND THEIR IMPLICATIONS

Theory Building as Selective Attention

T*he Structure of Scientific Revolutions* is the actual title of this seminal work by Thomas S. Kuhn (1962) because it is highly relevant to these lines of inquiry.

His essay elucidates the philosophical aspect of the development of ideas in the history of the sciences. He delineates normal from extraordinary science. Normal science proceeds slowly and rationally from one set of approved areas of inquiry to another—controlled by paradigms.

The field of extraordinary science does not reveal itself until the results of studies and intellectual inquiry have encountered difficulty with a system of ideas that cannot be resolved by the established means.

Normal science is conservative in nature; extraordinary science is more open-minded, much like our political representations of conservative, liberal, or progressive appellations. "Normal science forces nature into familiar conceptual boxes. . .the assumption that the scientific community knows what the world is like" (p. 24).

The paradigms Kuhn discusses are essentially filters that change reality and reassure us we are correct. A simple example from the field of psychology involves a set of trials in which subjects were provided with only brief exposures to playing cards (originally found in Bruner & Postman, 1949).

In these trials there were both normal cards—i.e., red hearts and black spades—and anomalous ones that had reversed colors and insignias, black hearts and red spades. Nevertheless, all subjects correctly identified all cards—but only insofar as the cards all "fit" their pre-conceptualized categories. The assumption was that the subjects made the red spades into black ones in spite of what they "saw" in reality.

In science it seems the same phenomenon occurs: We see what we are conditioned to see, test ideas that fit the paradigms we use and find the results we expect to find. Nor in this view of scientific behavior, Kuhn states, "do scientists normally aim to invent new theories and they are often intolerant of those invented by others" (Barber, 1961, pp. 596-602).

Even without proper paradigms to study nature, he notes, "In fact so general and close is the relation between qualitative paradigm and quantitative law that, since Galileo, such laws have often been correctly guessed with the aid of a paradigm years before apparatus could be designed for their experimental determination" (Kuhn, 1962, p. 29).

This has relevance for the "experimentally verifiable (EV)" view of cognitive theorists and practitioners to be discussed later. Because we cannot prove an idea or theorem does not make it untrue or, more importantly, unusable.

The application of this theorem involves all fields of inquiry, and certainly those in psychology. However, the main point regarding EV and psychological practice is that faith in our approaches, and resistance to change, may limit advances.

Theory Building As Selective Destruction
—The Leipzig Connection

Paolo Lionni wrote *The Leipzig Connection* (1993) to examine some of the changes in American education in the twentieth century. Wilhelm Wundt, a German experimental psychologist who had been the father of this field, influenced teachers by redefining education through laboratory experiences.

Earlier in the history of education, prevailing ideas involved those with historical roots in ancient Rome: "the drawing out of a person's innate talents and abilities by imparting the knowledge of languages, scientific reasoning, history, literature, rhetoric, etc." (p. 8).

For Wundt, "Learning is the result of modifiability in the paths of neural conduction. . .explanation of even such forms of learning as abstraction and generalization demand of the neurons only growth, excitability, conductivity, and modifiability. The mind is the connection-system of man and learning is the process of connecting." Lionni notes, "[Man] is his reactions" (p. 9).

Wundt's students became agents in proselytizing others into the new view of education by founding departments of education in the U.S. and other countries—an army at the ready.

One of Wundt's most influential students was Thorndike, whose views, according to Lionni, were "that man is an animal, that his actions are actually reactions, and that he can be studied in the laboratory" (p. 32).

While Thorndike believed in the singularity of environmental influence in all learning, and that a group of students who are taught the same information will differ only in their capacities, he later theorized these differences in learning were the result of "disabilities or deficiencies" and "that intelligence is set permanently before the student enters school" (p. 38).

Once again, it is instructive to see a theorist, in accounting for something that does not fit his paradigm, postulating a factor borrowed from an opposing system, that innate capacity, intelligence in this example, will make it work. If intelligence is a "given," as Thorndike assumes, then why persist with a system that is singularly environmental?

Since this early psychological formulation, later researchers have experimentally verified that intelligence is split between environmental and innate factors (see Hirsch, 1987).

It is not a fair criticism of Thorndike that he didn't anticipate this development, but his theory did not incorporate the divergence he noted, preferring instead to support ideas that seemed to be experimentally verifiable (EV) though at best incomplete or even wrong.

The major deficit in behaviorist formulations is their simplicity in representing the complexity of human behavior as we know it.

Although simpler behaviors can be explained with simpler theories, these theories could be incorporated into more complex ones, e.g.,..." psychoanalytic theory, which represents simple lower-level behaviors in primary-process thinking as well as more abstract secondary process ones." This formulation permits representation of both levels—closer to the complexity of humans as we know us (Rapaport, 1960, p. 30).

Lionni's central points are the modification of traditional forms of teaching through Wundt's experimental psychological ideas and the spread of these ideas that occurred at Columbia Teachers College with infusion of monetary support from John D. Rockefeller's enormous fortune.

The ideas were not just environmentally loaded, i.e., intended to control the masses, but presented as well to actively deride the "opposition," e.g., Dr. Maria Montessori's approach to aid the child's mind by changing the learning environment. "The result of Kilpatrick's diatribe was the suppression of the Montessori method in American education for the next fifty years. . .though they flourished elsewhere" (Lionni, 1993, p. 86).

It is instructive to note the nationalistic view of this debate—the Wundtian "Germanization" of education. Their paternalistic control of what were regarded as lesser peoples, counterpoised by others, specifically the Italian Montessori and later the Swiss Jean Piaget's evidence of the inheritance of cognitive structures.

"Wundt's influence led to H. H. Goddard, who invented the term 'Moron' and used psychological testing to prove the feeble-mindedness of great numbers of Jews, Italians, Hungarians, Russian and other Eastern Europeans attempting to emigrate to America" (Goddard, 1912, p. 104).

All that was required to pass on Wundt's thinking was to have a university—Teacher's College, New York City—and money. The money came from Rockefeller, a man whose wealth in 1910 was enormous, with assets of $800 million—valued at $19-plus billion today.

In an example of how extraordinary wealth affects psychological enterprises, when Rockefeller's fortune was being assailed he decided to make large donations to Columbia Teachers College to protect it.

"Through this 'education trust,' a virtually unlimited source of funds was made available to the Wundtian psychologists' ambitious designs on American education" (Lionni, 1993, p. 59). Wundt's ideas were spread by James McKeen Cattell, (of factor-analytic fame), G. Stanley Hall, and Edward Lee Thorndike, among others.

Wundt maintained, "Man is the summation of his experiences, of the stimuli which intrude upon his consciousness and unconsciousness," engaging stimulus-response psychology. (Lionni, p.7). This is an "outside-in" theory and, by definition, deemphasizes or replaces genetics and "inside-out" theories.

Noam Chomsky's inherited "transformational grammar" notions, in contrast to those of B. F. Skinner, were to be considered as well. This argument will be developed further, but it is worth noting the conflict between "inside-out" and "outside-in," the former representing insight theories, the latter those of the experimental and behaviorist fields, including cognitivists.

The spectrum of ideas and human experiences is replicated in all areas of life, including psychology. The experimentalist mindset is usually open to further testing of well-known postulates, while the clinical domain is mostly more open and humanistic. It should be noted the personal characteristics of both sets of practitioners differ in these ways as well.

Experimental approaches are easier to "prove" and attract adherents who may not be very aware of the limited underpinnings of their subject matter. Human behavior is far more complex than that evidenced in laboratory settings, requiring more sophisticated techniques and paradigms as well as experimentally controlled real-life behaviors.

This has implications for all areas of life, as noted earlier. The spectrum of human expression in phylogeny sets the stage for endless debates in human endeavors that are difficult to resolve and contain more heat than light.

Chapter Seventeen

THE HUMAN POLITICAL–PERSONALITY SPECTRUM

A MORE THOROUGH EXPOSITION of this spectrum can be found in an unpublished monograph of my own (Borelli, 2011). We are all born with personalities somewhere on this conservative–progressive spectrum, which accounts for an average expectable orientation in one direction or another. In essence—and this is important—we are all, in large measure, expressing our biology, not our psychology, when we express ideas.

This idea is similar to Freud's regarding the UCS and its influence in therapy and analysis, namely that the practitioner needed to be analyzed to adequately study psychoanalysis.

In the application of therapeutic change modalities, the nature (emotional balance and ability to relate) of the therapist is paramount. Essentially, the more behavioral the intervention (outside-in), the less crucial the therapist's nature is to the equation; the more reflective and analytic, the more crucial is the nature of the therapist's nature. I suggest re-reading this a couple of times.

Review—Theoretical Schema: Nominal, Ordinal, Interval And Ratio Scales

- Nominal
- Ordinal (Psychiatric Evaluations)
- Interval (Psychological Tests)
- Ratio (Future Models)

Theoretical Schema

These terms for various scales of measurement reflect increasing degrees of precision from *nominal* (just naming) through *ratio* (the most precise).

To use terms like "experimentally verifiable"(EV) is a broad exercise requiring more precision. Experimental psychologists, as others from traditional areas of science, have employed the terms above with good results.

If one places research from behavioral sciences on the N-O-I-R scale, it becomes clear they are functioning at different levels, and so are the mental health fields that employ them.

Psychiatry—apart from medical, organic science more broadly—is at best at the Ordinal level, as is some psychology, social work, and sociology. However, only psychological experimentation, intelligence testing, and some evaluation procedures are at the Interval level

One reason for the superiority of psychology can be found in the training of Ph.D. candidates, who must produce an original piece of research—a notion conspicuously absent from routine medical students' training.

The Psychological Field's Background

In the history of Psychology's precursor—philosophy—one must return to Plato's and Aristotle's divergent views. Plato believed that "reality does not reside in concrete objects but in abstract form represented in our mind." Aristotle believed, "Reality lies only in the concrete world of objects accessed through the senses."

What we have is "inside-out" thinking with Plato and "outside-in" with Aristotle. It is interesting that Psychology is still stuck with this dichotomy thousands of years later. Rationalism finds understanding in introspection, and Empiricism in observation of the external world. Later proponents included Descartes's Rationalism and Locke's Empiricism.

The Structure of Behaviorist Theory

Essentially there are three major types of behaviorism—early ones like Thorndike's SR, mediating (cognitive) ones like Osgood's, and the only one—Skinner's Operant Conditioning. There was also a theoretical attempt at rapprochement by Dollard and Miller to unite SR theory and psychoanalysis, but that will be discussed in a later chapter.

SR theories arose from the field of philosophy (Jacques Rousseau) and early psychology (Wilhelm Wundt). They assumed the organism learned primarily, or even totally, through brain excitation interacting with the environment.

A behavior was learned (reinforced) by a physical reward like food (e.g., Pavlov's Classical Conditioning), or emotion, like reduction of fear. These chains of learning/reward behaviors led to the compilation of larger behaviors, leading in turn, in their view, to the complexity of man.

Skinner's system was clearly behavioristic, even nihilistic, in its avoidance of anything not "psychological," so he pushed the behaviorist position to its logical end—literally. He avoided SR connections and instead postulated behavior, mostly from lab rats, that was "operant," that is, "operating on" its environment. The organism is behaving randomly, and when it is suddenly reinforced with a stimulus, it then learns what occurred just prior to the reinforcer, and that becomes part of its new repertoire.

This theory does not have the physiological reductionist position of other early behavioral formulations—for example, that food reduces the drive state of hunger—that relaxation reduces the drive state of anxiety. In Skinner's theory, the organism behaves mentally and not physically and, in so arguing, Skinner had enhanced an ultimate behaviorist "outside-in" position while making "outside" the priority. It may be instructive to note that his form of behaviorism has diminished over time—partly, or mostly, due to Chomsky's criticism of his language theory.

The Structure of Psychoanalytic Theory—Rapaport

David Rapaport was a mathematician and psychoanalyst who studied, and theorized about, psychoanalysis and psychology in general. One of his major works—*The Structure of Psychoanalytic Theory*—was published in 1960 for The American Psychological Association's series entitled *Psychology: A Study of a Science*.

In his review, Rapaport noted several theoretical constructs:

"· The subject matter of psychoanalysis is behavior—Empirical view

- Behavior is integrated & indivisible—Gestalt view
- No behavior stands in isolation—Organismic point of view
- All behavior is part of a genetic series—genetic view (not referring to physical, organic genetics as used today with DNA)
- The crucial determinant of behavior is the UCS—Topographic view
- The ultimate determiner of behavior equals Drives—Dynamic view, Nature and Nurture: Nature (Drives), Nurture (Drive objects)
- All behavior disposes of, and is regulated by, psychological energy—Economic view
- All behavior has structural determiners—Structural view
- All behavior is determined by reality—Adaptive view
- All behavior is socially determined" (pp. 39-62)

Rapaport's task, with the Ford Foundation's support, was to produce a set of ideas explaining what psychoanalysis is about. As with every discussion or set of ideas, it depends on the view of the person *with evidence marshaled in support* of that view. We must remember Rapaport's task was also to elucidate psychoanalysis, not argue with other theorists.

The italicized phrase above changes the focus from a person's bias to that person's view from within the scientific method—a very important difference. Without it, every discussion is only an opinion, and we humans are excellent at offering those.

Taking some of Rapaport's points one at a time:

- The subject matter of all psychologies is behavior.
- The Gestalt view is more reasonable, in my opinion, but not

one that is accepted by all psychologists or past philosophers.

- Behaviorists would argue this point, since they are "outside-in" theorists. The major issue here is not the difference in theory, which is very well known, but in how who we are—the type of brain we have—affects our views. So science clarifies views in a more objective manner but is not yet able to provide the "real" answer on this issue or others.
- The crucial determinant of behavior is the UCS. This statement is a problem for behaviorists and standard cognitivists, since for them it either doesn't exist or doesn't matter if it does. The central issue is that the cognitivists dumped the UCS to reduce the size and complexity of psychoanalysis. This achieved greater scientific proportions but ones less connected to the reality people see in their lives.
- The ultimate determiner of behavior is drives—a major tenet of psychoanalysis—but not for "outside-in" theorists; the most extreme opposition would come from Skinner.
- Psychoanalysis contains a theoretical device in positing primary-process functioning, which parallels learning theorists' concepts in the CS and secondary- process functioning that parallels cognitivists' abstract thinking. In this respect, psychoanalysis was closer to full human functioning, from its earliest versions.

The Structure of Cognitive Theory

Cognitive psychology belongs to the long tradition in thought of Empiricism and the dominance of the external world with "outside-in" learning. Lashley's (2007) research indicated that significant brain destruction did not affect learning. His student Hebb theorized that learning led to associations among neurons and cell assemblies. Cognitive psychology continued to receive support from academic studies that led to its being "experimentally verifiable."

To show how science proceeds—even EV science—Lashley deduced from his research on the destruction of large areas of rat brains that memory for maze running was retained, so he postulated that memory was stored everywhere in the brain.

Though he was correct in believing it was stored everywhere, he was wrong in the correlate—that the brain had no specialization areas. This error supported a cognitivist position anyway, and it took many decades before MRI scans corrected the error. So science does not follow a straight line of thought (think of Kuhn's work), though it eventually leads to more correct approximations of truth.

The first shift in thinking that led to the basis of cognitive psychology is the Plato–Aristotle shift that in turn led to Rationalism and Empiricism. The second shift, of academic/physiological studies, shone the spotlight on learning and paralleled learning theories in more mainstream psychology.

These shifts changed the conversation from how to study the mind to what the subject matter of the mind consisted of. In the process, then, of adopting a better, more accurate procedure, the procedure changed the conversation.

It provided the bifurcation of psychology's goals, which works, since learning and experiencing in a broader sense can co-exist;

however, cognitivists believed they had a procedure that explained all, or at least most, of human behavior—a sleight-of-hand maneuver.

As I explained earlier, Cognitivism changed the subject matter because it was easier to make psychology more of a science by reducing its scope, but should we accept this? No matter how experimentally valid the procedures and information obtained are, they don't change the notion that we have left a large area of human behavior unexamined.

Instead of viewing the difference between Rationalism and Empiricism merely as two schools of thought, perhaps the conversation should shift to how we have derived and maintained this difference in the first place.

My contribution to the discussion regards the type of brain involved. Rationalists are more dominant with, in the main, an emotional over intellectual balance, and Empiricists are more dominant with an intellectual over emotional balance. Rationalists may be those in the practice of psychoanalytic-type therapies and Empiricists more represented in cognitive–behavioral–experimental areas.

This may be a bit of a stretch, but the extrapolation can be legitimate that Rationalists share a great deal with those on the liberal end of the personal and political spectrum, and Empiricists with those on the conservative end of that spectrum. Think about this before you reject it out of hand simply because it is different.

An Alternative Approach to Theory and Treatment

The approach employed by most practitioners is a combination of medications and/or verbal therapy. Medications were created to turn on or turn off neuroreceptor and transmitter activity and thereby improve the symptoms of patients.

Therapy approaches attempted to deal with changing behaviors as well, but from the outside of course. The traditional types either remained the same and chose to apply techniques derived from neurotic non-using adults (analytic, behavioral, and cognitive), changed some aspects to accommodate differences (cognitive–behavioral–existential), or were supplanted by newer ones (therapeutic communities, historically).

To the extent the medications-and-therapy approaches remain separate and distinct, a less efficacious treatment regimen results. Of course, many therapy practitioners consult with medical psychiatric ones, but each of them may understand less than the desirable amount of information to progress in tandem.

Neuroreceptors and Transmitters

Julien (2016, p. 216) notes, "All our thoughts, actions, memories, and behaviors result from biochemical interactions that take place between neurons located in our central nervous system." The brain has billions of individual neurons, and some of them affect mood and cognition. Mood and motivation are mostly located in the amygdala, which is part of the limbic system.

When a neurotransmitter arrives at the synaptic cleft, it must be removed from the cleft or it will bind to the postsynaptic receptors. Every synapse is capable of removing the neurotransmitters from the synaptic cleft as an action to control drug effects.

For example, norepinephrine uptake is blocked by tricyclic antidepressants; serotonin uptake is blocked by serotonin-specific re-uptake inhibitor (SSRI) antidepressants, Dopamine uptake is blocked by Welbutrin, Zyban, cocaine, amphetamine, and methylphenidate.

Additionally, opioid analgesics and endorphins "exert presynaptic inhibition in the terminals of afferent sensory neurons to inhibit the release of pain-signaling neurotransmitters" (.p. 216).

Consider, in this context, the prevention paradox—the notion that binge drinkers are high risk and cause most of the damage to society, but that lower-level drinkers are less risk and cause less damage. Weitzman, Nelson, Rossow, and Romelsjo (2006) have demonstrated this is not true when the extent of damage is considered.

I am not concerned here with the very important public health implications, but with the paradox itself. In one respect, it may not be a paradox at all, because many instances of small damage can surpass a few instances of greater damage. Rather, it is the penchant for professionals in many fields to focus on "bright and shiny" objects, to the exclusion of other possibilities.

I believe this example illustrates the idea that assessment of more patients whom we think might not possess a target diagnosis is important, given the implications for those individuals and the larger society.

The authors point out the prevention paradox exists for tobacco, obesity, and injury as well. It relates to the issue in earlier assessment chapters of dealing with dysthymic and ADD populations, who don't seem to be at risk and who may not meet criteria and therefore have treatment withheld.

Analytic, Cognitive and Behavioristic Views from the 1950s

During the 1950s, psychology was dominated by behavioristic theories and experimentation from Pavlov and Thorndike and in the person of B.F. Skinner, who proposed a purer firm of behaviorism that had no role for "mind" (Aristotle).

Noam Chomsky was on the faculty of M.I.T. when, in 1959, he criticized Skinner's notion of mindlessness (Aristotle) and instead affirmed abstract representations within the mind (Plato).

Chomsky's view of language proposed an innate development and use of language expressed in his concept of Transformational Grammar (Chomsky, 1957). This concept argued that language develops from a subject's interaction with the environment whereby sentences lead to the development of other sentences generated by the subject's brain.

This critique, which received no response from Skinner, firmly established Chomsky as the premier linguistic theorist and, most importantly, aided the cognitive revolution that is now in its heyday.

Analytic and Cognitive Experimentation from the Present— Comparison, Resolution, and "Reframing" the Scientific Issue

It has become clear the EV definition of "cognitive" eludes clarity. However, when one adopts the Rapaportian structure of a complete theory, then it doesn't matter what we call these schools of thought, as long as we agree on similar terms and processes.

Unfortunately, the fields of psychology and other human behavioral sciences have seemed intent on at once re-inventing the wheel yet retaining their option of renaming and sometimes obfuscating. We have seen the UCS is the UCS even after co-opting it with a new name. The basis seems to be the utter refusal to yield anything to an opposing school of thought.

If we proceeded with a "new" comprehensive and clearly stated set of theoretical and therapeutic constructs, what would it look like?

The difference between psychology and other non-scientific fields, such as the chemical dependence field based upon the 12 Step Philosophy, is that experiments can be replicated and any changes be known and measured. However, if one has only "intuitions" and "hunches," no matter how much inter-rater agreement occurs, this is only a set of assumptions masquerading as science.

I do not mean to infer that only hard science can be permitted in discussions of human behavior, only that such ideas must be subject to scientific appraisal to be accepted in the larger treatment community. Prior to such evaluations, these ideas and assumptions can only have a heuristic value and allow some practitioners success in treatment and appraisal and in a very different field.

If CD practitioners always stay within the 12 Step Philosophy and accept its value in a dogmatic fashion simply because it has been around a long time, advanced ideas and techniques from scientifically derived fields can be rejected out of hand.

This is a dangerous and self-defeating mindset. Its conservative "purism" erodes into a stodgy and stale approach honoring past founders of a mostly humanistic and caring system.

Inpatient treatment staff advertise advances from medical and psychological fields, but the treatment process is often little changed. The field cannot pick and choose those approaches or ideas that "fit" what is already known. Scientists learn hard lessons about not falling in love only with comfortable ideas—it is only truth, trenchantly sought, that matters

---

Chapter Eighteen

"IS THERE IN QUANTIFICATION ALWAYS TRUTH?" THE COMPARISON, RESOLUTION, AND REFRAMING OF SCIENTIFIC ISSUES

A CLARION CALL FOR COGNITIVISTS is the phrase "experimentally verifiable treatment approach." The message is, "Don't rely on something that is not experimentally and quantitatively verifiable." This statement of pride and certainty has been a staple palliative throughout psychology's long history dating to the beginnings of experimental psychology and Wilhelm Wundt in the early 1800s, though even he might not have fully supported its validity.

It is sensible and reassuring to know something we do is "real," avoiding subjective states of mind in both the patient and therapist. So what is wrong with this proposal? In short, there are many propositions that are experimentally verifiable (EV) yet not true and, correspondingly, those that are not EV and still true—and useful.

The confidence cognitivists and other practitioners have in EV is based on a level of assumed precision that EV does possess but only in the areas it explores. Psychology has many similes that bear on this issue: Piaget's early work, and Skinner's Operant Conditioning, are two.

When Piaget hypothesized how a young infant or child's mind worked, experimentalists—notably in America—disparaged it as untestable. It was then, of course, as we have known for some time, but did its lack of quantification by methods drawn from experimental psychology of the time make it less true?

Correspondingly, did it become true only when its propositions were testable, though it worked? Montessori experienced the same skepticism from critics (see Thayer-Bacon, 2012, for an extended discussion of a trenchant "reframed" representation of Montessori's work).

A different example is Skinner's Operant Conditioning, which is not only EV but developed *de novo* from this Harvard psychologist's mind. It was, and probably still is, the most experimentally verifiable theory of human behavior in existence. However, did its verifiability make it truer? In other words, are there not bases for judging validity that do not employ formal statistics or EV?

An additional concern beyond EV is, is it *relevant*? In one experiment, a researcher dealt with schizophrenics and was able to get one or more subjects to ask for a stick of gum. This is experimentally verifiable, but to what end? Trivial research is useless by definition.

In Cognitive-Behavioral Treatment (CBT), when the technique of cognitive reframing is employed, does it merely objectify the quandary and leave the conflicted underpinning untouched? Further, for some theorists and practitioners, is there an underpinning—i.e., is there a UCS component?

For example, a patient of mine became unnerved by turmoil involving her teacher peers because it reminded her of verbal conflicts with her parents when she was a child. If this insight cognitively reframes the situation, so she now can control the situation via techniques, is the issue resolved?

The dilemma is that the reframing gave her temporary in-session control and relaxation, but the anxiety returned. What caused the continuance? Are we to assume reframing is insufficient as a cognitive approach, and that we require a better approach?

Do we assume a UCS aspect? If so, is that considered "cognitive"? Is it cognitive because it contains thoughts, since it also seems to contain emotions such as anxiety? Are feelings cognitions? If we are dealing with the UCS, why reject this psychoanalytic proposition? If "cognitive" treatment includes this, then maybe we are merely dealing with old psychoanalytic wine in new cognitivist bottles.

Chapter Nineteen

A ONCE-NEW APPROACH—A HYBRID OF PSYCHOANALYTIC AND COGNITIVE ELEMENTS

T HE PROBLEM, TO MY MIND, is the picking up and discarding of treatments and theories. There have been attempts to combine theories, e.g., Dollard and Miller with psycho-analysis and behaviorism, but these are the exception.

Dollard and Miller

Dollard and Miller (1941) dovetailed the theories of analyst Sigmund Freud and learning theorist Clark Hull. It is interesting to note that Dollard, an anthropologist, entered psychoanalysis at the Berlin Institute, and Neal Miller studied with Clark Hull.

They developed terms for the combination of physiological drive reduction on the one hand, and the mental states reflecting learned drives. They developed terms of:

- Approach–approach (attracted to two equally attractive goals)
- Approach–avoidance (attracted to and repelled by the same goal)

- Avoidance–avoidance (repelled by two equally unattractive goals)
- Approach gradient–avoidance gradient, reflecting degree of approach or avoidance states, and avoidance gradient steeper; i.e., the closer you came to the goal, the greater the resistance to proceed.

As to the resistance of theorists to welcome change, I believe this nihilistic approach is directly related to the narcissism of theorists and practitioners—"There shall be no other." If it were otherwise, the approach would proceed in more of the lockstep fashion of natural and physical sciences, retaining the old until it is disproven and then adding new insights and accomplishments.

My view combines the old and new, joining an older version of a more thorough therapy with a newer more effective one. As we have discussed, psychoanalysis—not known very well by practitioners in its heyday, and least of all today, is more thorough but with a few unwarranted assumptions, and sometimes takes excruciatingly long periods to effect change, if at all.

Its values are as follows:

Retaining the unconscious as primary. It recognizes that there is more to human behavior than meets the eye, as even lay people are well aware.

All psychoanalytic practitioners have not accepted the "eyes avoidant" therapy approach, but there clearly is a difference that should be explored. In my own practice, I long ago adopted it, and its opposite, and found it has the advantage of allowing patients to reflect on unconscious and pre-conscious areas of their life without the interruption of the therapist's watchful eyes.

Face-to-face therapy positions diminish this reflectivity. The reason for each approach is mainly that cognitive-behavioral practitioners do not wish to investigate the unconscious, while analytic practitioners do.

That avoiding the major source of human information is easier for EV-only practitioners is interesting, but not thorough and scientific; it is a way to partially deal with a problem by avoidance.

EMDR as Present-Day Psychoanalysis

This headline probably seems bold and unwarranted at first, but allow me to continue. EMDR is touted as an EV procedure and categorized as cognitive, though I don't see the cognitive-only description.

The procedure is of course designed to resolve traumatic issues cognitively and emotionally. The emotional component refers to the emotions aroused that are connected to the picture or target of the event.

However, there is more, in my opinion, in this procedure, and in those of some others. In the process of eliciting emotions, there are thoughts and emotions from the pre-conscious and unconscious areas of the brain. If one agrees with this, then EMDR lives on the border of the conscious and unconscious world.

My question is, how does this differ from the analytic process of revealing the unconscious that is associated with the patient's experiences?

More accurately, EMDR in the strict sense is for emotional reduction, specifically in traumatic or disturbed areas. However, it could also be employed as a simpler version of psychoanalytic treatment in both uncovering and resolving issues simultaneously, could it not?

I have also used the couch for relaxation and provide the patient with headphones via an extension cord, because it allows faster mind-clearing, which prompts associations.

Shapiro noted the saccadic eye movements in EMDR administration mimic the same movements in REM sleep. Robert Stickgold (2001, pp. 61-75) suggests, "The repetitive redirecting of attention in EMDR induces a neurobiological state similar to REM sleep [and] can then lead to a reduction in the strength of hippocampally-mediated episodic memories of the traumatic event."

Chapter Twenty

FORMAL ADDICTION THEORIES

Learning Theories

T O RETURN TO PAVLOV'S THEORY, the addict uses a drug that alters their need state by satiation. This alteration reinforces a future desire to return to that same state. Neither the AA/NA field nor Pavlov's theory knew that this process involved neurohormones and transmitter–receptor sites, because they had not yet been discovered.

Skinner's theoretical approach is quite different, in that physiological reductionism is not necessary; in this respect, his theory is purely psychological. He would believe the person has chemicals available in their environment and chances upon them when something is wrong that that chemical assuages. The "psychological" satisfaction then reinforces the habit to use (addiction).

Formal Addiction Theories—Robinson & Berridge

Robinson and Berridge (2003, pp. 25-53) composed a complicated and thorough analysis of addiction theories. This is the best single article I've ever read on the subject, and I offer their *Abstract* to inform:

"The development of addiction involves a transition from casual to compulsive patterns of drug use. This transition to addiction is accompanied by many drug-induced changes in the brain and associated changes in psychological functions. In this article we present a critical analysis of the major theoretical explanations of how drug-induced alterations in psychological function might cause a transition to addiction.

"These include (a) the traditional hedonic view that drug pleasure and subsequent unpleasant withdrawal symptoms are the chief causes of addiction; (b) the view that addiction is due to aberrant learning, especially the development of string stimulus response habits; (c) our incentive-sensitization view, which suggests that sensitization of a neural system that attributes incentive salience causes compulsive motivation or 'wanting' to take addictive drugs; and (d) the idea that dysfunction of frontal cortical systems, which normally regulate decision making and inhibitory control over behavior, leads to impaired judgment and impulsivity in addicts."

I believe you can see the headings employed cover the bases, and we need to know this material as well as our own terms. I have attempted to provide a truncated presentation of their ideas.

In their introduction, "Drug use does not inevitably lead to addiction. . .even though 90% have been exposed to a potentially addictive drug." The authors note that addictive drugs hijack neural circuitry involved in "pleasure, incentive motivation, and learning (residing) in the nucleus accumbens (Nacc)-related circuitry."

The oldest view of addiction is probably that drugs are pleasurable, and that repetition leads to tolerance and dependence; they are then continued to avoid the unpleasantness of withdrawal.

The Opponent Process Theory of Addiction is another version of this set of ideas. From the article, Solomon and Corbit (1973) posit an "a" process, an "A" related process, and a "b" process and "B" process, all of which reciprocate. It is too involved to proceed further.

Robinson and Berridge provide evidence that "conditioned feelings of withdrawal do not seem to be sufficiently strong or reliable to serve as the principal explanation for relapse."

Aberrant Learning. "Transition to addiction results from the ability of drugs to promote aberrant learning—associations more powerful than natural reward associations."

Explicit Learning. "Can vivid declarative memories even excessively optimistic or inaccurate memories, explain the transition to addiction; probably not. Instead they accurately predict drug pleasure and often agree their drug use is not justified by the pleasure they get."

Implicit Learning. These theories are S-R based and indicate over-learned habits become automatic and then compulsive. However, Robinson and Berridge counter, "Habit learning theories mistake automatic performance for motivational compulsion."

S-S Learning. "Drugs might distort the process by which the drug abuser connects a specific cue such as a particular place with drug-induced states." The claim of S-S theorists that "drug associated cues can engage brain motivational systems" seems to be too weak to be the basis for explaining addiction.

Incentive Sensitization. "The incentive-sensitization theory of

addiction focuses on how drug cues trigger excessive incentive motivation for drugs, leading to compulsive drug seeking, drug taking,
and relapse. . . . The central idea is that addictive drugs enduringly
alter Nacc-related brain systems that mediate a basic incentive-mo-
tivational function, the attribution of incentive salience.

"As a consequence, these neural circuits may become enduringly
hypersensitive (or 'sensitized') to specific drug effects and to drug-
associated stimuli (via activation by S-S associations). . .causing
pathological 'wanting' to take drugs . . .the sensitized neural system
responsible for excessive incentive salience can be disassociated
from neural systems that mediate the hedonic effects of drugs, how
much they are 'liked.'

"In other words, 'wanting' is not 'liking.' Susceptibility to sensitization is determined by a host of factors, including genes, sex
hormones, stress hormones, past trauma, etc., in addition to indi-
vidualized patterns of drug exposure.

"In summary, we suggest that at its heart, addiction is a disorder
of aberrant incentive motivation due to drug-induced sensitization
of neural systems that attribute salience to particular stimuli. It can
be triggered by drug cues as a learned motivational response of the
brain, but it is not a disorder of aberrant learning per se.

"Once it exists, sensitized 'wanting' may compel drug pursuit
whether or not an addict has any withdrawal symptoms at all. And
because incentive salience is distinct from pleasure or 'liking'
processes, sensitization gives impulsive drug 'wanting' an enduring
life of its own."

The quoted passages above allow you to hear, in their own
words, what Robinson and Berridge believe. The article continues

in great detail regarding how Skinner's operant conditioning and Pavlov's conditioned cues play a role.

This aspect of the discussion makes it clear that behaviors are "over-determined," as Erikson theorized. Secondarily, it demonstrates how earlier theoretical and experimental evidence continues to be wedded to later material—the advantage of science, which discards nothing in its quest for thoroughly ascertained truth.

A briefer and simpler exposition of these ideas can be found in McKim (1997).

Recent Developments—Parents of Millenials

The self-indulgent consuming society that has existed since the 1960s, at least, reflects individual narcissism as well as passive dependence. In earlier times, children were more active than now, and one could argue that this difference in level of activity is a simile for behavior change.

Passivity of individuals and groups, with its attendant lack of physical contact, leads to isolation of affect properly belonging in person-to-person interaction, with preference for an electronic means of communication, in general.

Today's youth and adults are rarely seen without one or more electronic devices in their very active hands—cell phoning, texting, e-mailing, face timing, IMing, Twittering, and web-surfing. Even members of Congress, who are very young in mind no matter their age, diminish the status of their office that they surrendered a long time ago to electronic communication.

Today's youth are less rarely, if at all, seen exercising or even moving significantly. The passivity and excess calories in their diets have led to them being the most obese children in history, even more than their thinner middle-age parents. Accompanying this physical change is illness—diabetes, hypertension, cancer, cardiac issues, etc.

Parents of Millenials

Besides weight gain, there is the problem of remote associating—dealing with people at a distance that may eventually not be satisfying to these younger people and will lead to more sterile relating and possibly greater reliance on chemical solutions.

Playing games on the Internet or video consoles is the new means by which people "entertain" themselves, continuing along the self-stimulation lines of chemical abuse–dependence.

Philosophical and psychological theorists are, as I have noted several times, far more sophisticated than any "theory" from AA/NA, even those who have proposed professional academic theories and treatments outside the AA/NA field. The major criticism in this regard is that those theories stick too closely to AA/NA thinking.

The same trajectory was followed by inpatient treatment from the past to the present—AA/NA was a decent starting place but never good enough to continue to the levels of the mental health field. Today's inpatient programs, and those in the recent past, have modified themselves to match what the mental health field was, and is, doing. It is as though mimicry is the highest form of flattery—and business acumen.

This includes medications and therapy approaches that were never a part of their field, which they have incorporated. It is laudable that the non-professional field incorporates superior approaches as they understand them, but where are their innovations?

If we begin our discussion with Pavlov's theory of a physiological reductionism that leads to reinforcement of behaviors, we will see an approach AA/NA used much later, perhaps without realizing it.

The addict ingests a drug, such as alcohol, in spite of corporate America's rebranding it as a legal one because of the number of "captains of industry" who have been addicted to it. Corporate America is almost always running such ad campaigns, which only serve to obfuscate the truth.

Chapter Twenty-One

THE HUMAN BRAIN SPECTRUM PROPOSAL

BELIEVE MOST PEOPLE THINK they have normal and typical brains of varying levels of intelligence, motivation, style, etc., and that specific or even general belief systems are learned, not inherited in any way (Borrelli, 2011). A portion of that article follows.

"A two-year-old girl dresses in her mother's accessories—high heels, beads, scarves. Women, while shopping, keep their carts close to them while men leave them at the ends of aisles. At construction sites, men peer endlessly through small cutouts on the wooden enclosure to observe machines going about their business, while women see no store to shop in and leave immediately.

"A husband and wife meet a five-year-old-girl and start talking with her. The husband asks how old she is, what school grade, and finally compliments her on a nice dress. At this point the 'interrogation' ends. His wife says, 'What a pretty dress you have. Did your mommy pick it, or did you choose it? I had a dress that color when I was your age. Well, your mommy must be a very good mommy, and I bet you are a very good girl.'

"Note the difference. The husband emphasizes information-gathering; his wife avoids this and goes straight to the relationship. This difference is probably not learned as an approach and has its source in conception. In the first year of life, a female infant can detect the presence of her mother in the room when she cannot see her. It will take a male child 2 to 3 months more to achieve this.

"Why? Her brain is wired for socialization, his is designed for information gathering with less emphasis on socialization. One wag has noted that men speak about 25 to 35 thousand words in a day, women about 45 to 55 thousand, with gusts up to 75 thousand. After he's spoken his complement for the day, he returns home, and she asks, 'What's new?'

"These gender differences are a few examples of psychology at work interacting with the environment, or are they? Were there training sessions or serious talks informing each group about what to do, or did they gravitate to the tasks, having a biological orientation to perform this way?

"One could agree they did gravitate, but that it was still learned behavior, because it is specific to the tasks at hand—all members of a society have similar enculturation—and that they merely express those similarities that were learned.

"But is it possible this is primarily the influence of our biology, specifically our brain types? This sort of thinking may be very foreign to most people's thinking, since we humans believe we learn everything, or almost everything. The notion of the *tabula rasa*—the Roman phrase for 'blank slate'—began the common-sense process of learning only, mainly from the outside.

"However, as time passes, scientific evidence reveals that biology is increasingly found to control those behaviors we once believed were learned. When I began to study psychology in college in the late Fifties, a schizophrenic child was believed to be the product of living with disturbed parents. Many years ago, it was already clear this was genetic programming at work and was not learned. The parents' genes were responsible, but not their observable behavior.

"Regarding politics, careers, and life in general, the idea that the brain exists to interact with an environment, and that the environment is separate from the brain, may be about as accurate as the notion that the Earth is the center of the universe, with the Sun and planets rotating around it.

"I believe the brain controls and contains everything—not everything we do or see, but the presence of *everything*. David Lanza and his co-author Bob Berman make this hypothesis clear in *Biocentrism* (2009). Even physics, which we ordinarily view as having immutable laws, is an illusion in some respects.

"In *Biocentrism*, Lanza and Berman present the Double Slit experiment as proof (2009, pp. 61-81). The experiment has two slits through which protons can enter—one on the left, and one on the right. Prior to this, physicists 'assumed that physical states existed before they are measured.'

"This discussion is very involved and should be read. In summary, objects can be waves or particles but not both. Yet when protons are fired toward the double slits, they change position depending on whether they are observed by a person.

"The protons can behave like waves or particles and, until they are 'shot,' their states of either are merely potential states. So, while the common man's view is 'a thing is a thing, the same thing no matter what,' this is clearly not the case.

"If the mathematical physical world behaves in strange ways, is it any surprise the mental world does also? That is, human existence is not as rigid and planned as some would like to believe. I draw your attention to the conservative mind's desire to see the world as conserved in always the same form.

"Thus, the challenge, in CD and other fields, is not only to provide evidence for a position but to present it in such a way as to aid resistant listeners to accept it.

"What I am positing applies to politics as well, of course. My view is that the political spectrum—from left (Progressive) to right (Conservative)—is not just a spectrum of ideas, but a spectrum of the brain's inherited tendencies projected onto the 'environment' with which it interacts. The Progressive to Conservative views are merely expressed by the choices we make directed by the brain types we possess.

"I am suggesting that brain type accounts for much if not most of the variance in behavior, in this case political behavior and its unpredictability, rather than to static factors like income level, attitudes in various areas of life, etc."

Politics As an Irrational Activity

Politics is often thought as a rational, brief activity— casting one's vote every so many years. However, this is not the case. It is fraught with as many pitfalls as other human activities.

The book *Political Animals* (Shenkman, 2016) was written to demonstrate, with evidence, the claim that politics is irrational. The book's cover has a monkey hanging from the letter "a" with a button that reads *I Voted*.

In the introduction Shenkman provides the example of shark attacks at the Jersey Shore, where Woodrow Wilson lived while President at the White House. When he ran for office a second time, he declared a "war on sharks," and this seemed to maintain his support from voters in those counties.

However, in the four counties where fear dominated, he lost 3 percent of the vote he had. In specific towns in those counties, the results were much worse. Nothing else could account for the difference except the shark attacks.

To make the comparison stronger, Shenkman notes, "The shark attacks in 1916 had the same effect on the voters of Spring Lake and Beach Haven that the Great Depression had on voters statewide in 1932.

"In 2000 George W. Bush and Al Gore vied for the presidency, and Gore lost only partly because of the Supreme Court's judgment but also because northern Florida had suffered an extreme drought. Research showed Gore voters voted for Bush, and that the tally amounted to thousands of votes. Since the election was decided by 537 votes, this was unbelievable but true" (p. xviii). Both these examples and others can be found in the book's introduction alone.

What we learn from this is that common sense is not common and not sensible. Westen's writings predate Shenkman's, but he is hardly mentioned in this text. It reminded me of a female journalist who capitalized on Erik Eriksen's theories of human development by presenting them in the popular press. Psychology and other fields are regularly co-opted by others. It occurs in the CD field as well.

Consider this:

1. Our brains do not make choices at the moment we think we have made them, but a full half second before we are conscious of making the choice. Further, experimenters could predict ten seconds before subjects performed an action, which hand they would move (Biocentrism). It would seem that selection tendencies are preprogrammed to respond to environmental alternatives—even those not seen before.

2. The ideas, institutions, structures—call them whatever you wish—are not separate from us but were created by the brains of people long before us, and still do, expressing their brains' predilections. Thus, those who come later in existence choose from the options that our brains are attracted to: The specific ideas and feelings evoked by those choices guide us. Of course, some brains were, and are, much more capable, and broaden the field of choices—they're owned by geniuses.

3. The brain influences events by *directing*, e.g., physical aspects like eye color and major illnesses, accounting for virtually all of the variance; by *orienting*—habits and attitudes; and by *influencing*, without accounting for all of the variance. In both events, the environment is never alone.

What relevance does this line of thinking possess for our area of inquiry? Essentially, it points to the fact that different brains interact differently with the same environmental events. Once one forgoes the idea that all brains are essentially the same and all environments have the same effect on those brains, one opens up a new world of ideas and beliefs.

In the case of addiction, we need to amplify our thinking to include this line of thought, in order to provide more accurate and complete theorizing and treatment. At present, it seems, treatment personnel of various stripes, professional and non-professional alike, do not employ such thinking or are not even aware of it.

Whether we speak of inpatient therapeutic communities or private practice treatment, assessment and therapy would change dramatically. I understand that practitioners may say they already see such differences among patients and residents and treat them accordingly; in fact, I suggest, they don't. The differences these practitioners have in mind typically involve character styles, sets of ideas, and so forth. While I agree these exist, it is not the static information possessed and employed by patients or residents that matters most in this approach—it is the manner in which the particular brain prefers to receive its information, and the manner in which it is employed.

The conservative mind is generally characterized as somewhat controlled, even rigid; it mostly prefers to hear what it agrees with; and, sometimes, that agreement can distort what a reasonable person would say.

I have had patients who were helped by therapy from professionals, including me, with EMDR that obviously changed their behavior for the first time in their lives. However, they then attributed the changes to techniques from groups they were part of at the time, like AA/NA, or to their own progress, but not EMDR!

An interesting relationship can develop between the patient who buys into this view of AA/NA, for example, and the recovering and other staff who view that as support for what they have done for the patient.

Additionally, it is difficult for any staff member to be balanced in a way that avoids ego inflation that cannot be part of effective treatment. Grandiosity is a more extreme instance of what can occur. This is another example of the need to know who you are—the *sine qua non* of all treatment.

Further, if one employs a more cognitive treatment that does not necessarily disagree with knowing oneself but emphasizes the technique as being much more valuable, it does diminish that dictum. Technique and personal awareness are not a 50–50 proposition.

The statement in the title of this volume—*The Match*—-is relevant here. Personal awareness is a minimal requirement in a therapist, but the "match" between the patient and therapist is very important, maybe in a paramount manner, in establishing and enhancing the therapeutic alliance. A therapist who works well with one group of patients will not necessarily work well with others because of this mismatch.

Further, the "match" does not primarily relate to issues like sharing a similar background to the patient in culture, use, age, education, gender, marital status, and such. It relates to the type of mind—its structure, flexibility, openness, acceptance, and tolerance of the patient's positions and values. In this respect the characteristics noted above may be helpful but much less important.

The Assessment Interview

The assessment interview involves many features—the more experience you have, the more you can ascertain. The most important aspect is you—who you are, and how well you know yourself. Besides skill with procedures, weakness in this area is the most important and potentially most limiting factor in a therapist.

The interview is, moreover, not only an information-gathering opportunity; it is a relationship opportunity. The difference between the two parallels the difference between men and women in their manner of relating to others, as you may recall from my earlier example.

Urinalysis. The intake process with CD people is the basic or advanced psychosocial alcohol/drug intake form(s). In the early days of assessment, the emphasis was on alcohol and drug data; around 1980, psychological and social elements were added as a reminder to obtain more about a person's life.

For many of us, it not only continued the process of structuring a more complete story but added elements that psychologists and psychiatrists, in the main, and other mental health professionals as well, had naturally plied in their work.

To those who arrived later in this broad field, it may seem surprising that the field of addiction only begrudgingly assented to this line of inquiry. The stumbling block was non-professionals following the tenets of drug-free approaches like AA/NA, as I mentioned in the introductory portion of this book, suggesting that it was the combined efforts of mental health professionals in not offering effective enough treatment to patients, try as they might, that led to this resistance.

It occurred in large part because those professionals did not understand addiction well or at all, and did not find it easy to relate to such patients, who were too different from their usual patient population. Specifically, CD people would be more likely to lie and manipulate, mainly out of a sense of inferiority, and not respect time, financial boundaries, or the duties of others.

Additionally, CD people sensed this discomfort as rejection, as well as knowing that the treatment, with or without medications, was not as useful as dealing with recovering people who could relate to their experiences and knew them so much better. The simpler AA/NA tenets worked in large part because those people believed what their sponsors and friends believed.

Besides this, one must pay obeisance to AA/NA free treatment anytime and anyplace in the world—no matter what condition you were in, and no matter how many times you failed—as long as you were willing to try again. This is powerful "medicine," and it made the CD person much more comfortable with the "fellowship" of such helping people.

So it took a great deal of time for the merging of recovering people and professionals. The process began with those of us who knew recovering people personally and also staffed the "schools" of addiction training in the 1970s in Princeton, New Jersey, and other places.

This in turn led to the formal certification process we know today. Those places of education allowed students who knew little or nothing about formal addiction principles, and others who knew little of real addicts' lives, to change their views.

There is a lesson to be learned here; being willing to confront issues separating us from each other parallels that of dealing with our clients/patients. How comfortable we are exposing our frailties determines how far we can travel in reaching people and changing them. Anxiety is often the precursor of change.

The Genogram

Information contained in the standard psychosocial interview is a beginning and maybe an ending, depending on where and whom you work for and how you define your task.

The genogram is the next very important format. It was first developed by psychiatrist Murray Bowen (1978) and enhanced by Monica McGoldrick and Randy Gerson (1985; third edition, 2007). It gave us a pictorial version of a family's history at a glance.

If you are unfamiliar with the genogram, it is worth your investigation. I teach, and have taught, in medical schools as well as engaging in private practice. In my lectures with psychiatrists, I introduce them to the genogram, since they are mostly unaware of it.

Once they understand the visuals and names employed, I ask them to obtain a genogram from an actual patient and not allow the rest of us to know who and what they are—not even their gender—though even this would be known in a "blind" study.

The rest of us then evaluate the four-generation family's relationships, mental and physical illnesses, personal histories, habits, and so on. In the process, we are able to ascertain the likelihood of the patient's gender and problems.

This exercise emphasizes the importance of one's past and gene influences. It moves the discussion mostly from psychology to biology, where it and the field are and should be today.

Since the genogram spotlights the past, it reinforces the view in many theories that the past is prologue—of paramount importance in assessing a person's life and difficulties.

It always seemed surprising that psychological and psychiatric theorizing have resisted the past as inconsequential in favor of the present. One possible move in that direction occurred with the emergence, years ago, of the cognitive movement, as I've mentioned before.

The experimental psychological movement decided not to pursue more complicated and difficult-to-validate psychoanalytic propositions. It was simpler to foster cognitive issues that were easier to replicate, and it therefore produced more effective treatments.

This makes sense, since we know what is gained, but what is lost?

One of the losses is a focus on the past in exchange for the immediate present. There is also the great assist from insurance companies that were enamored of quicker, cheaper treatment.

The major (and obvious) point about the genogram is its contribution to the family's past and the information required in assessment interviews to make a more complete diagnosis and treatment plan.

The Matrix

A "Matrix" is a representation of the dynamics of a patient presented in the same way as the genogram presented earlier in this volume.

Urinalysis

It is necessary to provide a urinalysis as well in order to be objective and fair with CD patients and, in some cases, with the person, professional, or agency that referred. It is possible but awkward to do so at a later time after you have come to know the patient well, and trust has been established to the point that to ask would violate a sensitive trust or seem inappropriate. In such situations, if a urinalysis is seen as the only way to prove the case, it is best to consider alternatives and check the S.O. or family members, or any others for whom the patient signed a release.

So, in the initial interview, a release is necessary, or the treatment will be rife with manipulation.

Therapy Choices

The assessment proposed above is quite effective. The choice of therapies is the next question, but, in the process, we must avoid narrowing choices. I believe most observers would agree that there are many choices—perhaps too many. The number of choices available is not the major concern I see; it is the number of choices a therapist employs or even can employ.

If most therapists choose some form of cognition, it may satisfy some that in so doing we have covered all the bases, but the spectrum of choices is not as broad as it seems if the hidden part of it is not among the candidates.

The primary thrust of this book is to present the long past in the field of psychology and its vast sophistication, compared to what is employed in other fields like AA/NA. The relationship is analogous to that in the spectrum I have just described. It is necessary, in my view, to have mental health practitioners who are knowledgeable and *skilled* in multiple approaches, not only *familiar* with them.

Psychoanalysis is a casualty of its own complicated theorizing and expense, but the former was and is critical, since Freud's theorizing is unparalleled in its explanatory ability.

Training in this field includes years of personal analysis. This is followed by years of training analysis—analysis of how one deals with patients, i.e., how one's own issues might get in the way of patient treatment, and attending classes in psychoanalytic theory and treatment at an institute—and paying for all of it.

Reasonable people would probably agree this is an exorbitant expense to incur in order to learn a treatment regimen that also is expensive for patients. When insurance payment is considered, it is worsened, because, while insurers do support this treatment, since all treatment is session limited (except bio-based diagnoses, for the most part), psychoanalysis will likely require more sessions.

It is surprising that insurance companies have a major influence in effecting what treatment is reimbursed and therefore chosen. It is the cost of therapy that limits a patient's choices—"I'll take whatever the insurance program pays for."

There are other patients who can pay out of pocket for sessions beyond what insurance allows, and they should have a choice of this approach. To be fair, there are quite a number of analytically trained people who are available, and I am not suggesting that practitioners entertain the full analytic experience of three times per week—leave it to those who have done so.

What *would* be useful is for practitioners to be analyzed—as patients. It aids everyone, no matter their chosen treatment field, since an examined psyche can only improve awareness. The reason is pretty straightforward: The psychoanalytic field requires a person to be treated in order to practice it, since one cannot analyze oneself.

I do not think the "supervision" of those seeking licensure by engaging in short-term treatment from a practitioner who had a similar therapeutic experience is in any way similar.

Other therapeutic choices are to be made by the future therapist, of course. That they will very likely choose some form of cognitive therapy is a given; what we have is what we will have—that is the way of the world. Cognitive therapy is not always, or mostly, the best choice. My point earlier reflects the multi-modal approach—that therapists are best off knowing a few therapeutic approaches.

Surprisingly, perhaps, I have heard many therapists offer some variant of, "I do my best to treat patients and only refer for a psychiatric evaluation when necessary."

The problem is that the decider's knowledge base is a biased format from which to consider alternatives. One aspect of that is mostly the therapist's emotional commitment to what they believe rather than a more objective assessment from a knowledgeable third party. Those of us who help people are connected to people by default and can become swayed by this.

A second likely area is not having a psychiatric consultant, or, worse yet, viewing psychiatry as a "last resort"—a term I've heard many times from social workers and counselors, though not typically from psychologists.

This is only surprising if one forgets that psychologists are closer in assessments and the role of brain-based behaviors common among psychiatrists than other mental health practitioners. Consequently, they are also more open to the idea of psychiatric referrals in general. This notion is related to brain-based behavioral controls and the role medications play.

The idea is not to refer when things have become very serious—this is Russian Roulette—but to view medication as a way to control symptoms, so therapy can work more effectively from early on.

We also need to consider the notion that medications complicate issues by diminishing, say, depression or anxiety, so the therapist cannot access them as well. This thinking was much more prominent in the early days of psychoanalysis. But in those days, medications were less effective, mostly because they were less targeted to relevant brain areas and therefore led to undesirable symptoms.

The major reason I have seen for the more recent reticence to refer usually involves counter-transference needs, expressed as a desire to continue working with verbal therapy; but to what end? Why make it harder to change someone more safely, not to allow their minds to function better and thereby make themselves better patients for psychotherapy?

It appears the medical–non-medical split among practitioners, as people, carries over to their professional roles. As noted in regard to different types of brain, which are in my view inherited. The social work–counseling group, in the main, is more likely to be verbal-supportive and less inclined toward numbers and brain physiology–chemistry.

Their experience, as is always the case, has proven to them that they were right and successful enough to help others. It is more comfortable and "natural" to proceed this way, so why add more complications with additional mental-health personnel and their side-effect medications?

We should, however, be accepting of alternate approaches and people to provide greater choice for a match to occur. Many of us have witnessed practitioners who were correct in their approach that led to mediocre results because the match was not also present.

Chapter Twenty-Two

MY IDEAL ASSESSMENT/TREATMENT FORMAT

TO CONTINUE FROM THE MATRIX PROFILE earlier, I practice counseling and therapy with an analytic bent because I was psychoanalyzed at Columbia in the 1960s, and my view of its benefits has already been detailed. I believe that analytic therapists are more liberal in orientation and of course brain type.

Over the years I have learned that cognitive approaches extinguish dysfunctional behaviors more quickly, so the roots of a deeper issue are more available to more extensive therapy.

I have also employed neuropsychological assessment via the Repeatable Battery for the Assessment of Neuropsychological Status (RBANS), along with interventions. This is not frequently employed by me, and when it is, I refer those with such issues to neuropsychologists, neurologists, and psychiatrists.

Additionally, I employ EMDR, also discussed earlier, in treatment to clear the path of traumatic experiences that block forward movement most of the time. CD people are particularly involved with trauma that leads to chemical use. This serves the purpose, of course, of alleviating symptoms but, unfortunately, then leads to habituation and another, more intractable problem.

EMDR treatment is more therapeutically useful than anything else I know of, though other treatments are also reported to work very well. But, since EMDR is opening up the mind and releasing UCS material to resolve trauma, it serves another purpose as well.

By decreasing or eliminating the affective component, it permits the trauma to move from STM to LTM and thereby become disengaged from regular mental and emotional intrusions.

In the process of trauma resolution, it also allows the Pre-CS/UCS material to present itself, which leads to release of very useful historical data that can enhance the psychosocial data as well. By definition, the patient may or may not be aware of this.

Many times as well, EMDR patients will spontaneously state: "I haven't thought of that in years" or "I never realized that." This information is usually germane to their core issues and fills out their history as a side benefit.

Subsequent to EMDR and some standard therapy one might wish to provide, I became aware of a new treatment in the summer of 2016. The Germans (Hasomed Corporation) spent twenty-five years developing this format, and the Pearson Corporation provides the licenses and training for RehaCom. It requires B level experience to purchase.

RehaCom consists of nine assessment modules such as Attention, Concentration, a variety of memory tests, and others. The focus is assessment and treatment of ADD, brain damage, and MS, etc.

After assessment is completed, even in part, the therapist moves on to the treatment modules, twenty-two of them, to expand the mind's ability to learn more efficiently. The modules won't permit advancing until the patient performs perfectly on lower-level modules.

As the patient succeeds in this endeavor, their brain changes their behavior. As an example, one male 24 year old, who had an extensive history of heroin addiction, had tried many treatment approaches. These included multiple outpatient, inpatient, detox, and drug-free chemical types, and the family had given up hope.

I employed EMDR and RehaCom, and his parents were impressed with the results, since they included the pattern of multi-level aspects of addiction to be treated. He had been diagnosed with ADD, and was on medication for it, had difficulty focusing, and also drove like a maniac at high speeds in a powerful car.

Within a month or so, he was much more capable of focusing on computer materials like architectural designs and reading books and newspapers. His driving had also changed remarkably, in no longer having the urge to speed or become upset in the process. He discontinued the ADD medication for a time to prove he did not need it, and did so twice.

The general format for my approach is to assess the primary and secondary diagnoses and then refer for a psychiatric evaluation for medications. Since he was active with heroin, Naltrexone (in the form of Vivitrol) was employed, as well as the ADD medication.

I began with verbal therapy and, mainly, EMDR, since emotions play a significant role in driving thoughts. In his case, trauma needed to be resolved before more focused work could be done. Subsequently, RehaCom was used to change his brain's thinking and habits, and that worked better than I thought it would—I'd had no experience with this to know either way.

Another patient in his twenties was severely ADHD and anxious. He made progress when I first saw him in his late teens to resolve his having found his mother's dead body at age 14 after she suffered from alcoholism of a heritable type and her relatives were alcoholic as well.

When I saw him, I was not certified for EMDR but referred him to a practitioner, and after about a year with some success, his recovering alcoholic relative convinced him to follow AA treatment instead.

He returned recently, and I employed EMDR and tried to move him to RehaCom an in attempt to resolve his ADHD as I had with the prior patient. He abhorred medications and preferred not to ingest any, but after a couple of sessions his anxiety bled into his functioning.

I switched to using the Color Relax CD as he lay on the couch in a relaxed position with the direction to lie there after the Color Relax was done and to try to sleep. From the very first session he was impressed with his relaxed state and with feeling so good he wished he could "feel this way all the time."

I told him he could by lying down at home and playing my recording of the Color Relax. I followed this up, and his relaxation was lasting. At this point I will go further to prepare him for RehaCom to change the issues he wanted changed, like his ADHD and impulsivity.

In the fifty years I have been practicing, I have only known medication as the most effective way out of this conundrum, though I tried others. With RehaCom there is another very effective way that is also drug-free. I do not wish to overreach by singing Reha-Com's praises on the basis of a small N of several cases. However, it is a good start, and passing on the word of this approach seems wise and helpful.

The Order of Therapies with Complex Patients— A Case Study

A patient of mine in pre-EMDR and pre-RehaCom days was a middle-aged male with strong addictions. He used an "8 ball" of cocaine and had sex with a woman whom he was either dating or paying for, on a daily basis. He thought this was a great plan, since whenever he passed away, he would be happy.

His issues included addiction—cocaine and alcohol—severe ADHD, narcissism, owing ten years of IRS returns, and financial issues with others, as well as being unable to pay my fees, having dysfunctional family problems with his wife and only child (his wife had divorced him by the time I saw him), and, later on, his allergic reaction to all ADD medications prescribed by his addictions psychiatrist.

I suspect there are therapists who would have chosen a different order of interventions, based upon their training and experience, that might work as well or better than mine did with this patient.

My approach has always been to first control the addiction and co-occurring disorder, simultaneously with supportive therapy, merely to keep a patient involved and motivated until the medications began to take effect. You can see that drug-free practitioners would not employ medications and would possibly prefer group and individual counseling and therapy. The "outside in" is king, and conscious cognitive learning—lecturing—is the correct approach.

Once medications reach a therapeutic dosage, the psychiatrist, with input from me, settled on the dosage. Although I had begun verbal therapy before this point, the next order of business was a choice of one or more specific areas for change.

The patient's failure to file IRS returns was a dangerous risk for him, since he could have been fined and charged with violating the law at any time, but he wanted to leave it alone.

His finances needed repair, and at points in his life he had made about $1 million per year; this was not the case now. The medications and therapy alleviated his anxiety and confusion enough for him to focus on his business.

His inability to pay me would require my referring him elsewhere or delaying payment to me, and I always choose the latter. If therapists are financially unable to wait for their money, the choice is made for them. If they are financially stable, as I was, then the choice is refer or wait, and I waited.

Once this first issue is resolved, a second is the therapist's rigidity about rules and/or his or her own level of personality resistance. My view has always been that some patients cannot do what is "right" because of life circumstances, and that their need for help outweighs my need for income or time.

In fact, the patient I have been describing ran up a bill of $7,000.00 to $8,000.00 at two different times, and paid the total each time. The ability, or willingness, of a therapist to allow for such delays in payment, I might add, fosters a stronger relationship with the patient, and it did with ours.

I would suggest a therapist consider this possibility in their future and be prepared to make a choice, perhaps before therapy even begins—a simpler solution than waiting until therapy is under way.

This patient's dysfunctional family could, moreover, wait until he was more integrated, because I investigated the extent of the problem with his ex-wife and son. Although he protested a great deal about how difficult she was to live with, her view was the reverse, and his son agreed. The son used the "f" word repeatedly, as his father did with us and, later, in family therapy with his father.

The wife and son were not only functioning well without him, they were resistant to engaging with him. The decision to avoid including them was appropriate, and, much later, when he was more stabilized, the family was more open to engaging with him because he had improved and genuinely wanted their love and forgiveness.

After six months or so, the psychiatrist could not find a non-allergic medication for his ADHD. In retrospect, if I had had RehaCom and EMDR, the lack of a medication would have been far less of a handicap.

This case demonstrates one of the major aspects of my treatment regimen—resolving as many issues in the whole of his life as possible. To do less is to invite relapses under stress. Thus, one cannot be satisfied with abstinence or resolution of immediate family resolutions; the patient's world is much larger than that.

Here's a medical metaphor that demonstrates problem resolution pre- and post-medical discovery. I know of a family in which one adult male member died from a bacterial infection before the discovery of penicillin, while his brother lived because penicillin had by then become available: Timing can sometimes be literally everything.

Continuance of therapy involved couch and face-to-face work with both cognitive and analytic approaches. The end result for the patient was many months of abstinence from cocaine and alcohol, his backup drug.

Relationships with his wife and son led to a cease-fire, and he moved on with his S.O., who had been with him initially and referred him to me.

And a serendipitous, even astounding event capped his achievement. My remembrance of it is as follows: He and his S.O. moved into an apartment in a raised ranch. There were two other buildings on that property, a small cottage and a large house with federal designation as a protected property.

An older woman tended to the flowers and shrubs there, and she shared a pleasant very friendly relationship with the patient and his S.O. Over time, they learned that the woman was the owner of this property and of another large home with federal designation as well.

The woman eventually approached them about giving them the property with the three homes, and revealed that her nephew had inherited the other large house. She was offering the properties for free, since she had no other relatives.

They couldn't immediately accept the offer, though, since the town and state hired lawyers and psychiatrists to verify the woman's capacity to consummate the transaction. After months of investigation, they agreed she was legally and psychiatrically competent, and the couple could take possession after her passing—timing!

Different Medications in Different Patterns

To review: About 1980, I spoke with psychiatrists about changing the standard mix of medicines and therapy, including verbal and analytic types; and anti-depressant, anxiolytic, ADD, and brain-based types like Symmetrel (Amantadine Hydrochloride), an NMDA receptor antagonist.

This profile was different, since it modified mood- disordered and cognitive functions, along with medications that addressed specific chemical drugs of abuse. Symmetrel had mixed success but opened the field to a major change, in my opinion, with other similar medications of the new class.

In the same period, Narcan made its appearance as an opioid antagonist. Both of these medicines opposed the effects of the targeted drugs of abuse.

Narcan was so powerful in its remediation of states of unconsciousness, or even coma, that, when an addict came to the ER in such a state, an injection of Narcan led to rapid clarity. The addict felt very angry and even explosive—as though they had experienced a pleasant dream that had dissipated immediately.

When the opiate attaches itself to relevant neuroreceptors, it will last until a person has metabolized it. In extreme instances, it could lead to coma and death before such metabolism is completed. Narcan immediately erased the opioid from its neuroreceptors, leading to a clearer and healthier level of functioning.

Additional medications included Naltrexone, a milder version of Narcan, as an oral version, and later, as an injectable version, Vivitrol IM, lasting three to four weeks.

Antipsychotic formats began with anti-seizure medications,

Neurontin, then Depakote, then Abilify (oral) and Maintena (Abil-ify-IM), then Latuda. Maintena permits patients to receive benefits when they are non-compliant with medication regimens, because, as an IM medicine, it is part of the patient's system and cannot be undone.

Non-compliance is one of the main reasons why patients of all types say, "The medication isn't working."

The GENOMIND approach was mentioned under the Psychi-atry heading in the chapter on Evaluating Clinical Comparisons. This genetic advance makes the medication choice a clearer and more objective process and reinforces psychiatry's role in symptom mediation.

Psychiatry has advanced via Genomind, factor analysis, and personality clusters, as well as through improved medications. The entire fields of medicine, mental health, and so on are seeing great advances. The human Genome Project has changed approaches to CD people, but it has worked backward to intrauterine techniques as well.

Multiplying the Effect

In the CD field and many others, the best treatment services are provided by individuals who are often high-priced as well. The goal here, in my view, is to multiply the effect of one person helping one person, or, for example, one person helping a small number of pa-tients in a group.

There is a way to replicate what clinical psychology did many years ago. In the early twentieth century, the Rorschach was taught as a one-on-one process, because it required intense observation and complicated scoring—a situation that still exists today, except in the later procedure of employing a different set of ink blots with a group of patients.

It is possible to do so today—not with the Rorschach, which is passé, having been superseded by the MMPI and PEP-Q, for example; my view is the PEP-Q, based on Cattell's factor analytic approach, provides different information in its machine scoring but is more practical as well than the MMPI.

These tests are given to one person at a time, but also to many individually in groups. There are other excellent, and even superb, instruments that could be adapted for groups as well.

Regarding the RehaCom, I wish to make it clear this was not designed to evaluate more than one person at a time and with more than one examiner at a time. The German researchers, who developed it over a twenty-five-year period, designed it this way.

I employ the test in the required manner, not in the theoretically possible manner I will present now. I offer it here merely as a possibility for consideration.

RehaCom is an instrument to assess the mind's functions in the assessment modules and then challenge it to expand and change. The mental process of "changing the mind" I presented earlier in this volume is paralleled here.

Since RehaCom has an educational nature to it, it might be provided in individual PCs one-on-one in a group monitored by one or more therapists, and could multiply the effect, of course.

In inpatient CD settings the staff, often composed of recovering people, have a noble and satisfying role in "therapizing" their charges. However, if we are interested in helping more people more quickly and effectively, then new solutions are needed.

It is possible for counselors and therapists to move patients toward abstinence and more effective living. However, what they do is not always consistent and effective. A program like RehaCom is both consistent and effective, and its ability to be administered in a group—even a large group—is valuable.

Additionally, unlike staff, it has a procedure that, in my opinion, laser-focuses on changing minds in precise ways. By comparison, analytic therapy can bring a patient to emotional insights but does so slowly and sometimes not at all. EMDR does it more quickly and effectively. The process being discussed here is the same as the Rorschach, PEP-Q, and MMPI having been "multiplied."

Alfred A. Borrelli

Chapter Twenty-Three

THE PRESENT GENERATION

THE SELF-INDULGENT, CONSUMER-DRIVEN SOCIETY that has existed since the 1960s at least reflects individual narcissism as well as passive dependence. In earlier times, children were more active than they are now, and one could argue that this difference in level of activity is a simile` for behavior change.

Passivity of individuals and groups, and lack of physical contact, lead to isolation of affect properly belonging within person-to-person interaction, in preference for an electronic means of communication, in general.

Today's youth and adults are rarely seen without one or more electronic devices in their very active hands—cell-phoning, texting, e-mailing, face timing, IMing, twittering, Snap-Chat and web-surfing.

They are rarely, if at all, seen exercising or even moving significantly. The passivity and excess calories have led to the most obese children in history, even more than their thinner and healthier parents. Accompanying this physical change is illness—diabetes, hypertension, cancer, cardiac issues, etc.

The passivity and sense of anomie it produces is anathema to avoiding CD and other mental issues. *Activity* is critical—don't watch sports, participate; don't e-mail or use other electronic procedures, write words and meet people. Consider buying products from brick-and-mortar places and not solely, or at all, on the Internet. Humans don't relate well at a distance.

The question to ask of these young people is, "How often in a day do you have direct, involved contact with others? How many of those people are other than your close friends? How many of all your contacts are Internet 'friends'?"

Consider different styles of parenting examples: In a café I saw a child about two years of age quietly sitting and feeding herself with contentment, without demands from parents who obviously loved her and responded periodically.

Correspondingly, a boy in a restaurant with his parents and grandparents was eating in their presence, but not *with* them. Their non-responses to him, and his isolated feelings, were obvious. He ate in a lonely, mildly sad, fashion.

When he finished, he had an electronic game with him and began playing it. In the 45 minutes my wife and I were there, no one at the table had any interaction with him. Is it any wonder that some children lean so heavily on self-stimulation? Chemicals are a wonderful palliative—for a short while.

Parents thus play a significant role, but they often represent a group called "helicopter parents" who hover over their children. Several years ago, *60 Minutes* interviewed Millennials and asked questions like, "You have a good-paying job, and like the work and your co-workers and administrators. If the company around the corner would pay you a little more, would you go?" They said they would; it is loyalty to self, engendered by the God Narcissus, whom their parents know well.

This *60 Minutes* segment was modified and repeated a few years later, with the same result. It should come as no surprise, if you remember that the parents are also part of a particular generation—postwar baby-boomers who wished to provide their children with the experiences and "things" they themselves did not have.

These parents also changed their parental role dramatically—they wished to be their children's "peers and friends." The plan was to push their children to work harder and join more groups, to pave the way for them to attend Harvard and Yale and be loved by their offspring.

In my experience, these parents are also more accepting of casual CD use, probably due to the parents' own use in their development. They also engage in "means–ends" thinking or quid pro quo—if you don't get something, don't give something. It changes a more human relationship into a business relationship.

About two years ago, I read about a young Mexican college student who had saved as much money as he could each year and in the end spent it all on one thing—the cost of one college course! Such passion! Such discipline!

Older, more mature parents would be proud of this child, but I immediately thought of what Millennials themselves would think before knowing. A gift for myself, a good time, an electronic device, a newer model iPhone?

Phrases from the 21st Century

> "Internetese": *LOL* (Laugh out loud); *OMG* (Oh, my
> god); *ROFL* (Rolling on the floor laughing); *YOLO*
> (You only live once); *Where you at?* (not proper English).
>
> *I'll refer you back.* (The Latin word *ferre* means "to send," and
> adding "re" is therefore unnecessary
>
> *Wrecking havoc*—Wreaking havoc
>
> *Close proximity*—(proximal *means* "close")

Internetese has corrupted language and young people now speak in a type of Morse Code. Speaking leads to abbreviated thinking and, consequently, a changed perception of the world.

Hyperbole: words reserved for outstanding events or ideas on a rare basis are now used frequently, e.g., that was an "amazing" taco/dessert/person.

"Dude" and "cool" are of questionable use and are much older terms from the Old West and Black musicians from the Twenties, which young people probably don't know. "History is now."

Texting leads to hand and wrist injuries.

In the 1990s I heard a phrase used for the first time by adults— "going forward." An initial thought is commonsensical—in what other direction could you go?

Another overworked phrase is "Having said that." This merely states a situation in which we all know you said it, so why repeat it? My point is, language now unnecessarily states the trite and re-dundant, and since language reflects our environment (think the Sapir-Whorf Hypothesis), it would seem we are as confused as it is.

Dating in groups: For several years now, when a couple wishes to be exclusive, they still "date," but within a large group; what is its purpose, to resist the process of being intimate and separate, as seems to be required by typical development here in the West?

As employees in stores, they are abrupt and inappropriately casual with customers; it is as though they are being imposed upon and only work because they need money and/or their parents made them work.

Commitments are not what they were; superficial relationships can easily be broken. Millennials who should vote don't, because they are above the "corrupt and immoral process" and will not participate, even though they will suffer in the outcome.

Young Hollywood actors speak about their "craft" as though they were already accomplished. The older and accomplished actress Lauren Bacall responded to a younger actress, who had described herself as a "legend," by remarking, "She's too young to be a legend."

Superheroes: In the past, less sophisticated programs were the result of lesser technology, mediocre acting, and storytelling. Today, superheroes are more extreme—can fly without a device, are immune to injury, can grow instantly to enormous size, etc. The games played are just as unrealistic and lead to unrealistic expectations. In the past, seeing a movie was simpler, and when kids left the theater, they left the movie behind. Today, with unrealistic games, the movie continues. Adding mind-altering drugs enhances this unreality.

Parental Role

"Those who cannot remember the past," Santayana warned, "are condemned to repeat it." Besides the helicopter parents who want their kids to have and do everything, there is the role of the environment. We all are surrounded by an environment that can powerfully influence our behavior and each of us from different generations—not the I-Phone "quickie generations" that may last ten years, but the standard twenty-five-year ones representing a person's ability to develop and then reproduce themselves.

Having lived a long life and experienced many situations, I have a somewhat different view of life and its influence. I was born before World War II, and it left me with a sense of caution—not fear, but a seriousness toward life. During and after the war people realized how close they came to having everything collapse in terrible ways, like having Adolf Hitler as the world's leader.

When G.I.s returned home, they married, purchased homes, and had kids with a sense of exuberance and satisfaction. Their children incorporated their parents' values of being thankful for what they had. Some of the parents had parents who had lived through the Great Depression, and also realized how life can change in dramatic and terrible ways.

The impact of this war and others modified people's views of life in ways that those who came later did not experience. Some or most of us, as their children, had incorporated these lessons and values and passed them on to our children, who are now in *their* fifties and early sixties.

However, some of our children heard the situations we lived through but were not changed as we were—why? I believe it is because they did not live through a war, in this case. Am I suggesting children *need* a war? Absolutely not, but they do need environmental pressures that lead to a similar result.

For example, did your children work as adolescents; were they required to serve others in ongoing tasks, even those within the house; did they do so consistently; did they earn and save money; did they learn to be less self-centered; did they share?

These ideas are a superficial representation of the person–environment relationship. There is a more involved representation—the interaction of brain types with environments in dynamic ways, which is relevant here, but it is a topic for another time.

Another part of the influencing environment is education, especially the part omitted—geography and civics. Students in the past twenty to thirty years don't know much about where countries, states, and cities are located. Even more importantly, they are ignorant of the definitions of Communism, Fascism, Capitalism (in its many forms), Libertarianism, and Socialism which they think is like, or the same as, Communism.

These young people are not alone; they are accompanied by their "teachers"—parents, journalists, politicians, entertainment figures, etc. In fact the odds are that those reading this book don't have accurate knowledge of such matters either.

There is a book called *Today's Isms* that defines all this extremely well. It was first published in 1954 by William Ebenstein, and "Today's" refers to the time when the subject was a hot topic; the latest edition was published in 1993.

Chapter Twenty-four

"FUTURE SHOCK"—HOW LONG DO WE HAVE TO WAIT?

T HIS IS THE LAMENT OF THOSE BORN later than the 1950s especially, who have grown accustomed to "having" things and obtaining them quickly. In this regard, think of parents who provide their primary-grade children with computers and cellphones so they might have a "better life." At this time Silicon Valley engineers and scientists won't permit their children to attend schools that provide calculators.

Besides the contribution of ADD and impulsivity as psychiatric characteristics, the main mover is the fantastic rate of change—of planned obsolescence. This is the process of making products that are designed to fail within a short period of time, so we must purchase replacements.

So not only children but "adults" need to jump on this roller coaster to fill their relatively empty lives—bereft of serious relationships—with excitement, with things.

There are those of us who are much older and willing to wait, and think, and choose carefully, but the deeper issue for our society is Toffler's ideas, as brilliant today as they were in the 1970s.

Genetics control part of the equation of "nature vs. nurture," but as we can see, in this conundrum nurture holds sway unless parents are willing to attempt to push back against the tide of the "rush," a word used to describe a type of addictive drug effect—interesting!

So, the question for your child(ren) and yourself is, at what pace do you and they "move"?

The title of this chapter duplicates that of a book by Alvin Toffler. "Toffler argued that society is undergoing an enormous structural change, a revolution from an industrial society to a 'super-industrial society'. He believed the accelerated rate of technological and social change left people disconnected and suffering from 'shattering stress and disorientation'"—future shocked.

"The urban population doubles every eleven years, the overall production of goods and services doubles each fifty years in developed countries" (Wikipedia).

Toffler noted our society began by making non-durable products, and this reflected the end of durable products and practices—family, religion, physical nature of towns, etc.

I have thought about Future Shock, not only with regard to today's children as well as those in past decades, but especially to those from pre- and post-World War II. We are different from those who came much later, and perhaps it is related strongly to us being much less future shocked.

I.P. Treatment Program Dynamics

Young people mostly, in I.P. treatment programs, are like the little boy I described—with identity issues, isolation, seeking love, and mentoring. The staff and residents are also similar, sometimes regardless of their ages.

In many visits to I.P. programs, I have observed those who love to play the role of a "guru" like Yoda of *Star Wars* fame. One presumes they seek validation, even from their charges, and that this leads to quick and intense rapport and identification, whether it is appropriate or not.

The question I have is, would a guru play this role if he or she were psychoanalyzed or at least in competent therapy?

At this point the CD field has more sophisticated approaches everywhere—AA/NA, verbal therapies accompanied by trauma resolution, and ones that unblock areas of functioning so other therapies can work more efficiently.

It is very reasonable to expect medicines will improve, becoming even more targeted by way of receptor interaction, with fewer or even no side effects. In all of these advances we can be sure AA/NA treatment facilities in the main will mimic the major fields in order to be more effective and competitive.

As always, there will continue to be some facilities and groups that maintain the drug-is-a-drug theme that stridently refuses to modernize, even as it expresses a nonsensical view. The opposing trend of being open-minded waits upon more individuals who possess a different brain type as well as better education in scientific ways.

It is most important to remember the main fields of addiction—medical and psychological—that have made the advances others follow. In this regard, state-of-the-art developments in medical fields already in existence presage changes some of us have looked forward to for many years.

The neonatal field has performed surgical procedures in utero since about 1980 (The Human Genome Project, 2011) and provided medicine infusions to prevent inherited diseases. Surgeries include repairing bladder obstructions, tumors, spina bifida and neural tube defects, and cancers, among others.

Those inherited diseases that cannot be dealt with via surgery are more complicated, in my opinion, because they await research in genetic formulations—medicines that will be introduced to the fetus via a bacterium that will travel through the bloodstream and switch things on and off in the brain. At present they include Duchene muscular dystrophy, retinoblastoma, and cystic fibrosis, among others.

Compare the great efforts of scientists and therapists in dealing with addictions in the distant past with more recent developments. In large part, the Human Genome Project (2011) in the 1990s led to enormous and unprecedented leaps in new ideas and approaches.

The promise of the genetic approach—note GENOMIND introduced earlier—is fantastic compared to present-day verbal and AA/NA approaches.

My strident response is not meant to be disparaging, only realistic. For a CD person, relative, or acquaintance, these older, more rigid approaches are delaying the best treatment available to those who are suffering. The question is, does the CD person, or do significant others, wish to seek out someone who wants to engage in the verbal-only approach?

In my long years of practice, this desire is occasionally what people wish, and that is their right, but I am overwhelmingly asked to provide the most effective and quickest treatment I know of. The majority of patients, and their significant others, need to know differences among treatments, and then choose.

When those of us who use advanced techniques that have experimentally validated support, especially when medications are involved, others tend to deride our approach. The people who react this way include AA/NA or professional verbal-only therapists.

I view the AA/NA resistance as a combination of honest preference for an approach that has saved lives and mostly saved greater degradation and grief for them and their families, as well as that of others. This is an admirable goal—honesty always is—even when it leads to problems for those needing assistance.

The remainder are mostly those who believe they and others in the fellowship must stand together against those trying to dismantle a noble and time-honored "treatment." One more extreme and dangerous example follows.

I treated a twenty-four year-old male many years ago who had a primary heroin use history with occasional use of mood-altering and hallucinogenic street drugs. His co-occurring disorder was severe ADHD and borderline functioning.

Some examples from his life include the following. He had a great number of tattoos, and one day he severely burned his abdomen, which also had tattoos. The burns were third degree, and he treated the pain with opiates. He rejected out of hand my recommendation he go to the ER.

On another occasion he was traveling into town from a job site and saw an attractive woman. He beeped his horn at her, and she smiled and waved. This suggested to him he should send her flowers, so he could date her; he saw no problem with this.

He owned an expensive car with a bent frame that greatly lowered its value. His plan was to create a serious accident to "total" the car. He would hit a concrete blockade in front of the New Jersey Turnpike tollbooths. I asked whether he had thought of how he was risking his life, but he was confident he could survive.

I present his psychiatric history as a prelude to what occurred in his NA group at that time. Those in the meeting thought the multiple medicines he was ingesting caused problems and told him to discontinue them, "To see who the real *you* is."

Once off the medications, he did not tell me about this plan until afterward, as I recall; he behaved bizarrely in his acting-out, but we were able to reestablish his more stable functioning level.

The surprising part is that the NA group members, in their grandiosity, presumed they knew better than us professionals, especially since the AA/NA hierarchy had stated in their bylaws that those in the group are not professionals and should not interfere with professional treatment.

So the future of CD treatment requires more honest brokering among all treatment providers. To describe an alternate approach in disparaging and even dishonest ways is deceitful and damaging, and indicates that you view the alternate approaches as threatening and even superior, which they very well may be.

A SUMMARY NOTE

I HAVE COME TO THE END of this eleven-year project and, though I have more to say, it is time to end. My hope in writing this book has been to pass on most of what I have learned in the past fifty years and hope it galvanizes new practitioners to keep their minds as open as they can in the process of trying new approaches.

It is worth hoping for more effective change in mental health fields of theory and treatment—a change that relegates human behavior to a status worthy of the complexity we all see, but which has been trivialized by those interested in quantification at any cost, in their rush to mimic the physical sciences.

What we have seen via theories, experimentation, and real life is that the past is prologue. More importantly, genes and their primordial progenitors continue unabated in their inexorable quest to direct behavior toward *their* pre-ordained ends, as we humans revel in the "freedom of our choices."

REFERENCES

Adams, E.W. (1966). On the Nature and Purpose of Measurement. *Synthese, 16*, 125-169.

Ansbacher, H.L., & Ansbacher, R.R. (1956). *The Individual Psychology of Alfred Adler.* New York: Harper Torch Books.

Allport, G.W., & Odbert, H.S. (1937). Trait Names: A Psycho-Lexical Study. *Psychological Monographs, 47*, 211.

Amana, T., & Toichi, M. (2014). Effectiveness of the On-the-Spot EMDR Method for the Treatment of Behavioral Symptoms in Patients with Severe Dementia. *Journal of EMDR Practice & Research, 8*(2), 50-65.

Astrachan, B.M. (1970). Towards a Social Systems Model of Therapeutic Groups. *Social Psychiatry, 5*, 110-119

Bandura, A. (1978). *Social Learning Theory.* New York: General Learning Press.

Bandura, A. (1973). *Aggression: A Social Learning Analysis.* Englewood Cliffs, NJ: Prentice Hall.

Barber, B. (1961). Resistance by Scientists to Scientific Discovery. *Science, 134*, 596-602

Benson, H. (1984). *Beyond the Relaxation Response.* New York: Berkley Publishing.

Bion, W.R. (1959). *Experiences in Groups.* New York: Basic Books.

Blais, M. (1997). Clinician Rating of the Five-Factor Model of Personality and the DSM-V Personality Disorders. *Journal of Nervous and Mental Disease, 185*(6), 388-394.

Borrelli, A. (2011). *How Much Biology Is In Your Psychology?* Unpublished manuscript.

Boring, E.G. (1929). *A History of Experimental Psychology* (2nd ed.). New York: Appleton-Century-Crofts.

Bowen, M. (1978). (Genogram). Genopro.com.

Brett, G.S. (1912). *A History of Psychology* (Vol. 1). London: George

Allen and Unwin.

Briggs, K.C., & Briggs, I. (1998). *MBTI Handbook: A Guide to the Development and Use of the Myers-Briggs Type Indicator* (3rd ed.). Washington, DC: Consulting Psychologists Press.

Bruner, J., & Postman, L. (1949). On the Perception of Incongruity: A Paradigm. *Journal of Personality, 18,* 206-223.

Bugental, J.F.T. (1965). *The Search for Authenticity* (sub. ed.). New York: Holt, Rinehart & Winston.

Buss, D.M. (1995). A New Paradigm for Psychological Science. *Psychological Inquiry, 6,* 1-31.

Carlson, J.F., Geisinger, K.F., & Jonson, J.L. (Eds.). (2017). *Buros Mental Measurements Yearbook.* Lincoln, NE: University of Nebraska Press.

Cattell, R. (1957). *Personality & Motivation Structure and Measurement.* New York: World Books.

Chomsky, N. (1965). *Aspects of the Theory of Syntax.* Cambridge, MA: MIT Press.

Chomsky, N. (1957). Generative Grammar. In N. Chomsky, *Syntactic Structures* (pp. 1-162). Cambridge, MA: MIT Press.

Cozolino, L. (2002). *The Neuroscience of Psychotherapy.* New York: W.W. Norton.

DeLeon, G. (2000). *Therapeutic Communities: Theory, Model and Method.* New York: Springer.

DeYoung, C. (2006). Higher-Order Factors of the Big Five in a Multi-Informant Sample. *Journal of Personality and Social Psychology, 91*(6), pp.1138-1151.

Diagnostic and Statistical Manual of Mental Disorders, DSM-V (5th ed.). (2015). Arlington, VA: American Psychiatric Association.

Diagnostic and Statistical Manual of Mental Disorders, Text Revision (DSM-IV-TR) (4th ed.). (1994). Arlington, VA: American Psychiatric Association.

Dole, V., & Nyswander, M. (1967). Heroin addiction: A Metabolic Disease. *Archives of Internal Medicine, 12,* 98.

Dollard, J., & Miller, N.E. (1941). *Social Learning and Imitation.* New Haven, CT: Yale University Press.

Ebenstein, W., Ebenstein, A., & Fogelman, E. (1999). *Today's Isms: Socialism, Capitalism, Fascism, Communism and Libertarianism* (11th ed.). New York: Pearson.

Embedded Figures Test. (1969). Washington, DC: Consulting Psychologists Press.

Erikson, E. (1953). *Childhood and Society.* New York: Triple Bookkeeping / Norton Press.

"Ethanol History-From Alcohol to Car Fuel." ethanolhistory.com

Ewen, R.B. (2010). *An Introduction to Theories of Personality.* New York: Psychology Press.

Eysenck, H.J. (1993). Creativity and Personality: Suggestions for a Theory. *Psychological Inquiry, 4,* 147-178.

Fancher, R.E., & Rutherford, A. (2012). The Sensing and Perceiving Mind. In R.E. Fancher & A. Rutherford, *Pioneers of Psychology: A History* (4th ed., pp. 167-171). New York: W.W. Norton.

Fillmore, M.T. (2003). Drug Abuse as a Problem of Impaired Control. *Behavioral and Cognitive Neuroscience Reviews, 2,* 179.

Foa, E.B. (1979). Failure in Treatment of Obsessive-Compulsives. *Behaviour Research and Therapy, 17,* 169-176.

Frager, R. & Fadiman, J. (1998). *Horney and Humanistic Psychoanalysis: Personality and Personal Growth* (4th ed.). New York: Pearson Longman.

Frances, A. (2013). *Essentials of Psychiatric Diagnosis.* New York: Guilford Press.

Frances, A., & First, M.B. (2000). *Am I Okay? A Layman's Guide to the Psychiatrist's Bible.* New York: Random House.

Friedman, M., & Rosenman, R.H. (2004). Type A and B. *Clinical Cardiology, 27,* 308-309.

Freud, S. (1913). *Interpretation of Dreams.* New York: Macmillan.

Galton, F. (1941). Measurement of Character. In W. Dennis (Ed.), *Readings in General Psychology* (pp. 435-444). New York: Prentice Hall.

GENOMIND, genomind.com

Goddard, H.H. (1912). *The Kallikak Family: A Study in the Heredity of Feeble-mindedness.* New York: Macmillan.

Goldberg, L.R. (1993). The Structure of Phenotypic Personality Traits. *American Psychologist, 48,* 26-34.

Goldberg, L.R. (1992). The Development of Markers for the Big Five Factor Structure. *Psychological Assessment, 4*(1) 26-42

Jha, A. (2013, November 10). Heisenberg's Uncertainty Principle. Science. *The Guardian,* p. 1.

Hirsch, E.D. (1987). *Cultural Literacy.* Boston, MA: Houghton Mifflin.

Holland, J. (1973). *Making Vocational Choices: A Theory of Careers.* Englewood Cliffs, NJ: Prentice Hall.

Horney, K. (1950). *Neurosis and Human Growth: The Struggle Toward Self Realization.* New York: W.W. Norton.

Jacoby, R. (1983). *The Repression of Psychoanalysis: Otto Fenichel and the Political Freudians.* Chicago, IL: University of Chicago Press.

Johnson, B.A., & Ait-Daoud, N. (1999). Medications To Treat Alcohol. *Alcohol Research and Health, 23*(2), 99-105.

Julien, R. (2016). *A Primer of Drug Action.* New York: Worth.

Jung, C. (1923). *Psychological Types.* New York: Harcourt & Brace.

Kelly, G. (1955). *The Psychology of Personal Constructs* (2 vols.). New York: W.W. Norton

Klein, D.B. (1970). *A History of Scientific Psychology: Its Origins.* New York: Basic Books.

Klein, M. (1960). *Our Adult World and Its Roots in Infancy: Human Relations* (Tavistock pamphlet #2). London: Tavistock Publications.

Kohlberg, L. (1984). *The Psychology of Moral Development: The Nature and Validity of Moral Stages, Essays of Moral Development* (Vol. 2). New York: Harper & Row.

Kuhn, T. (1962). *The Structure of Scientific Revolutions.* Chicago, IL: University of Chicago Press

Langs, R. (2004). *Fundamentals of Adaptive Psychotherapy and Counseling.* Basingstoke, UK: Palgrave Macmillan.

Langs, R. (1989). *Rating your Psychotherapist* (Vol.1). New York: Ballantine Books, p. 175

Langs, R. (1988). *Decoding Your Dreams.* New York: Ballantine Books.

Lanza, R., & Berman, B. (2009). *Biocentrism.* Dallas, TX: Ben Bella Books.

Lashley, K. (2007). *Intropsych.com/ch06__ memory/lashleys_ research.html.*

Lionni, P. (1993). *The Leipzig Connection.* Sheraton, OR: Heron Books.

Reik, T. (1983). *Listening With The Third Ear: The Inner Experience of a Psychoanalyst.* New York: Farrar, Strauss & Giroux.

Livesley, W.J. (2001). *Handbook of Personality Disorders.* New York: Guilford Press.

London, P. (1964). *Modes and Morals of Psychotherapy.* Florence, KY: Taylor & Francis.

Maslow, A. (1943). A Theory of Human Motivation. *Psychological Review, 50*(4), 370-396.

Mazzola, A., & Lopez, V. (2009). EMDR in the Treatment of Chronic Pain. *Journal of EMDR Practice and Research, 3*(2), 75.

McGoldrick, M., & Gerson, R. (2007). *Genograms: Assessment and Intervention* (3rd ed.). New York: W.W. Norton.

McKay, M., & Fanning, P. (1986). Progressive Relaxation and Breathing. new harbinger.com

McKim (1997). *Drugs and Behavior* (6th ed.). Englewood Cliffs, NJ: Prentice Hall.

Mead, M. (1928). *Coming of Age in Samoa.* New York: William Morrow.

Myers Briggs Personality Test. The Myers & Briggs Foundation.com

Michel, J. (1986). Measurement Scales and Statistics: A Clash of Paradigms. *Psychological Bulletin, 3*, 398-407.

Mischel, J. (1968). *Personality and Assessment.* New York: Wiley.

Mischel W., & Ayduk, O. (2004). Willpower and a Cognitive-Affective: The Dynamics of Delay of Gratification Affective Processing System. In R.F. Baumeister & K.D. Vohs (Eds.), *Handbook of Self-Regulation: Research and Theory.* New York: Guilford Press.

Mischel, W., & Rodriguez, M.L. (1989). Delay of Gratification in Children. *Science, 244*, 933-938.

Mischel, W., & Shoda, Y. (1995). Cognitive-affective Personality System. *Psychological Review, 102*(2) 246-268.

Moont, R., Pud, D., Sprecher, E., Sarvit, G., & Yarnitsky, D. (2010). Distraction. *Science Direct, 150*(1), 113-120.

Neurotek.com

Pavlov, I.P. (1927). *Conditioned Reflexes: An Investigation of the Physiological Activity of the Cerebral Cortex* (G.V. Anrep, Ed. & Trans.). London: Oxford University Press.

Harman, H. (1976) *Modern Factor Analysis* (3rd ed., rev.). Chicago, IL: University of Chicago Press.

Randolph, C. (1998). *RBANS (Repeatable Battery for the Assessment of Neuropsychological Status).* Bloomington, IN: Pearson Publishing.

Rapaport, D. (1960). *The Structure of Psychoanalysis Psychological Issues.* New York: International Universities Press.

Rauch, S., Defever, A.M., Favorite, E., Garrity, T.C., Martis, B., & Liberzon, I. (2009). Prolonged Exposure for PTSD in a Veterans Health Administration PTSD Clinic. *Journal of Traumatic Stress, 22*(10), 60-64.

Reik, T. (1983). *Listening with the Third Ear.* New York: Farrar, Strauss & Giroux.

Rehacom. (2016, August). Software Program. New York: Pearson.

Robinson, T., & Berridge, K.C. (2003). Addiction. *Annual Review of Psychology, 54*, 25-53.

Rogers, C. (1961). *On Becoming a Person.* New York: Houghton Mifflin.

Rogers, C. (1959). *Psychology: A Study of a Science* (S. Koch, Series Ed., Vol. 3, pp. 184-256). New York: McGraw Hill.

Rogers, C. (1951). *Client-Centered Therapy.* Cambridge. MA: The Riverside Press.

Rogers, S., & Silver, S.M. (2001). Is EMDR an Exposure Therapy? *Journal of Clinical Psychology, 58,* 43-59.

Rose, G. (1981). Strategy of Prevention: Lessons from Cardiovascular Disease. *British Medical Journal, 282,* 1847-1851.

Rozeboom, W.W. (1966). *Scaling Theory and the Nature of Measurement.* Cham, Switzerland: Springer International Publishing.

Santayana, J. Brainyquote.com

Samuel, D., & Widiger, T. (2008). *A Meta Analytic Review.*

Saulsman, L., & Page, A. (2004). The Five Factor Model and Personality Empirical Literature: A Meta-Analytic Review. *Clinical Psychology Review, 23,* 1055-1085.

Schafer, R. (1954). *Psychoanalytic Interpretation in Rorschach Testing.* New York: Grune & Stratton.

Schore, A.N. (1997). Mind In The Making: Attachment, The Self-Organizing Brain, and Developmentally-Oriented Psychoanalytic Psychotherapy. *Journal of the American Psychoanalytic Association, 45,* 841-867.

Shapiro, E. R., & Carr, W. (2012). An Introduction to Tavistock-Style Group Relations Conference Learning. *Organizational and Social Dynamics, 12*(1), 70-80.

Shapiro, F. (1995). *Eye Movement Desensitization and Reprocessing, Protocols and Procedures: Basic Principles.* New York: Guilford Press.

Shenkman, R. (2016). *Political Animals.* New York: Basic Books.

Sixteen Personality Factor Questionnaire (16 PF, 5th ed.). (1993). Champaign, IL: IPAT Corp.

Skinner, B.F. (1938). *The Behavior of Organisms.* Cambridge, MA: The

B.F. Skinner Foundation.

Snow, R.E., & Marshall J.F. (1987). *Conative and Affective Process Analysis*. Hillsdale, NJ: Lawrence Erlbaum Associates.

Spencer, H. (1975). *The Relaxation Response*. New York: Berkley Publishing.

Stevens, S.S. (1946). On the Theory of Scales of Measurement. *Science, 103*(2684), 677-680.

Stevens, S.S. (1951). Mathematics, Measurement and Psychophysics. In S.S. Stevens (Ed.), *Handbook of Experimental Psychology* (pp. 1-49). New York: Wiley.

Stickgold, R. (2001). A Putative Neurobiological Mechanism of Action. *Journal of Clinical Psychology, 58*(1), 61-75.

Straley, J. (2014). It Took a Eugenicist to Come up with 'Moron', Code Switch. http://www.npr.org/sections/codeswitch/2014/ 2/10/ 267 561895/it-took-a-eugenicist-to-come-up-with-moron, p. 1.

Terwilliger, R.F. (1968). *Meaning and Mind*. London: Oxford University Press.

Thayer-Bacon, B. (2012). Maria Montessori, John Dewey, and William H. Kilpatrick. *Education and Culture, 28*(1), 3-20.

The Human Genome Project. www.genome.gov/pages/ research/ dir/nhgrintramuralbrochure2011.pdf

Sullivan, H.S., Gawel, M.L., & Swick, H. (2008). *The Interpersonal Theory of Psychiatry*. New York: W.W. Norton.

Thorndike, E. (1932). *The Fundamentals of Learning*. New York: AMS Press.

Toffler, A. (1970). *Future Shock*. New York: Random House.

Wechsler IQ Tests, Psychological Corporation, now owned by Pearson Publishing, New York, with different dates for each version at each age level.

Weitzman, E., Nelson, T.F., Rossow, I., & Romelsjo, A. (2006). The Prevention Paradox. *Addiction, 101*(2), 295-296.

Westen, D. (2008). *The Political Brain*. New York: Perseus.

Wilson, B., & Shoemaker, S. (1992). *The Big Book* (4th ed.). New York: Alcoholics Anonymous World Services.

Winter, D. (2013). Still Radical after All These Years: George Kelly's "The Psychology of Personal Constructs." *Clinical Child Psychology and Psychiatry, 18*(2), pp. 276-283

Witkin, H., Karp, S., & Goodenough, D. (1962). *Psychological Differentiation.* New York: Wiley.

Wolpe, J. (1958). *Psychotherapy by Reciprocal Inhibition.* Palo Alto, CA: Stanford University Press.

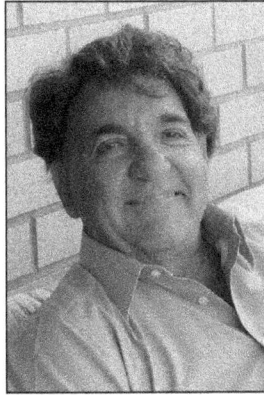

ABOUT THE AUTHOR

Alfred A. Borrelli has a B.A. and M.A. in Psychology and completed all coursework only for the Ph.D. in Psychology at the Graduate Faculty of New School for Social Research. He is licensed as an L.P.C. (Licensed Professional Counselor) and L.M.H.C. (Licensed Mental Health Counselor). He spent 800 hours in psychoanalytic psychotherapy at Columbia University with Anthony F. Philip, Ph.D., A.B.P.P., for a period of six and a half years. He has taught at the City College of New York, New York Medical College, UMDNJ (University of Medicine and Dentistry of New Jersey), and Bergen Regional Medical Center.

As Clinical Psychologist and Clinical Director at the New Jersey Regional Drug Abuse Agency (Liberty Village)—Inpatient Treatment for 250 residents in three facilities, he introduced dramatic changes in the treatment model that had only recovering people "treating" residents. He has spoken at national and international conferences as well as having been the guest professional on The Montel Williams Show on the occasion of the death of actor River Phoenix.

He has been in the psychology field for fifty years and has evaluated and treated tens of thousands patients while working for institutions and agencies on all phases of chemical dependence treatment, as well as treating patients with other psychiatric diagnoses. He developed a treatment format that included changing the patient's brain with medications and paralleling this with intensive individual treatment.

Al Borrelli maintains a private practice in Saddle Brook, New Jersey, and New York City.

www.ingramcontent.com/pod-product-compliance
Lightning Source LLC
Chambersburg PA
CBHW022348280326
41935CB00007B/121